Mental handicap
in the community

Mental handicap in the community

Edited by
Alan Leighton

Foreword by
Sir Brian Rix, CBE, DL, Chairman, MENCAP

Woodhead–Faulkner

New York London Toronto Sydney Tokyo

Published by Woodhead–Faulkner Limited,
Simon & Schuster International Group,
Fitzwilliam House, 32 Trumpington Street,
Cambridge CB2 1QY, England.

First published 1988

© Alan Leighton 1988

British Library Cataloguing in Publication Data
Mental handicap in the community
    1. Great Britain. Welfare services for
    mentally handicapped persons.
    I. Leighton, Alan
    362.3'8'0941

ISBN 0-85941-447-7

Designed by Ron Jones
Typeset by Goodfellow & Egan, Cambridge
Printed in Great Britain by Billings and Sons Ltd, Worcester

Contents

Contents

Contents

Foreword

The Royal Commission Report in 1957, which led to the Mental Health Act 1959, recommended a shift in responsibility for mentally handicapped people from hospitals to the community. After more than thirty years, this has still not been fully achieved. Even for those mentally handicapped people who have been transferred to life in the community, we remain concerned that there are, in many cases, inadequate support services.

Some eight years ago, when I was appointed Secretary General of MENCAP and in reference to the need for increased partnership between statutory and voluntary sectors and the 1971 White Paper *Better Services for the Mentally Handicapped*, I remarked, 'But above all, what we are looking for is *action*, as to how to make existing services better. We have been patient long enough'. The contributors to this book, all experts in their own field, illustrate that whilst much has been achieved, much remains to be done. In welcoming this publication, I hope those of you who read it will be inspired to further the aims of care in the community.

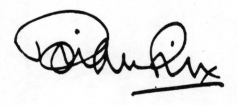

Sir Brian Rix, CBE, DL
Chairman, Royal Society for Mentally Handicapped Children and Adults

The contributors

Andy Alaszewski is Senior Lecturer in Health and Social Policy at the University of Hull. He has been involved since 1972 in research on the development of policies and services for people with a mental handicap. His doctoral thesis 'Institutional Care and the Mentally Handicapped' (University of Cambridge) was published by Croom Helm in 1986. A revised edition of a survey of services for mothers with a mentally handicapped child, which he undertook with Sam Ayer, 'Community Care and the Mentally Handicapped', was also published by Croom Helm in 1986. He is currently completing a major study, funded by the DHSS, into the development of an alternative model of care for children with a profound mental handicap. This is to be published by Croom Helm (A. Alaszewski and B. N. Ong (eds.)) and called 'Residential Care for Mentally Handicapped Children'.

Chris Bailey commenced his career with people with learning difficulties in 1976 after working for seven years in the commercial sector. He started as Industrial Unit Instructor for an Adult Training Centre in East London, qualifying as a teacher for people with a mental handicap in 1978, writing a thesis on employment and the mentally handicapped under the guidance of David Norris at the Dorset Institute of Higher Education.

Since 1978 Chris Bailey has gained considerable experience in negotiating, placing and supporting people with a wide range of abilities, but concentrating on those people with more severe disabilities, in their training, work experience and employment options.

At present he is developing new employment initiatives within Ellingham, providing an employment agency enhancing clients' opportunities to work in the community, together with discussing future day care provisions.

Ann Brechin trained as a psychologist at Aberdeen and Nottingham

Universities working at first with families and self-help groups in a community setting, and later as a Senior Clinical Psychologist at Charing Cross Hospital and Great Ormond Street. For the past eight years she has been a lecturer with the Health and Social Welfare Department of The Open University, involved most recently in collaboration with MENCAP in the development of the course, 'Mental Handicap: Patterns for Living'.

J. E. Buggy is a specialist Senior Social Worker with Manchester City Council.

James Cummings retired after 25 years as Director of MENCAP's Education, Training and Employment Department. Trained originally as a social worker, he worked for some years in the field before training in the early 1950s as a teacher of mentally handicapped children. He worked for several years in Israel and has undertaken Unesco and other international consultancies.

Mary Dalgleish, from a background in developmental psychology, was commissioned by the DHSS Works Group over several years to look at the effects of environmental design on services for people with mental handicaps in various development project areas.

Peter Farrell has been co-tutor to the MSC Educational Training Course at the University of Manchester since September 1977. He also works as an educational psychologist in Manchester LEA where he specialises in working with children with severe learning difficulties, their families and teachers. He has a number of workshops for teachers and parents on behaviour problems, classroom management and behavioural teaching techniques. He is also familiar with the effects of recent legislation on the assessment and placement of children with special educational needs.

Michael Gunn has been a Lecturer in Law at the University of Nottingham since 1978. He has a keen interest in the law as it affects people with mental handicap. This interest has resulted in contributions to conferences, courses and some writings. He also has developed an interest in mental health law and criminal law.

Fred Heddell has for four years been the Director of Education, Training and Employment Services for MENCAP – the Royal Society for Mentally Handicapped Children and Adults. Prior to joining MENCAP, he was Head Teacher of Warren Special School in Lowestoft, and has for more than 20 years taught in schools for children with learning difficulties and mental handicaps. He is also known for his work and writing on a number of television series, including *Let's Go*, *Accident at Birth*, *With a Little Help from the Chip* and currently *A Life of Our Own*.

Dr Seamus Hegarty is Deputy Director at the National Foundation for Educational Research in England and Wales. He has done research and published widely on special needs education. He has a particular interest in educational integration and wrote the overview volume to the 20-book series on special needs in ordinary schools published by Cassell. He is editor of the *European Journal of Special Needs Education*.

Dr James Hogg is Reader and Deputy Director in the Hester Adrian Research Centre, university of Manchester. He has been carrying out research in the field of mental handicap for the past 20 years. At present, his major areas of interest are ageing and mental handicap, and profound retardation and multiple handicap. Work in the latter area is being undertaken in collaboration with MENCAP's Profound Retardation and Multiple Handicap Project. Dr Hogg has written and edited six books concerned with these subjects as well as more general publications dealing with assessments and staff training. His scientific research has appeared in both British and American Journals.

Dr A. Holland is Senior Lecturer and Honorary Consultant Psychiatrist at Bethlem Royal Hospital.

Loretto Lambe is co-ordinator of the MENCAP PRMH project.

Alan Leighton is Consultant Group Director, Marketing and Communications, MENCAP, and is a self-employed writer, broadcaster, scriptwriter and television interviewer. He is also a Justice of Peace and a Director of a number of companies concerned with the welfare of people with a mental handicap.

Tom McLean, MBE, has been Director of Nursing Services Calderstones since 1972 and a Registered Mental Handicap Nurse since 1962. He was appointed Unit Director of Nursing Services for the Brockhall and Calderstones Mental Handicap Unit when these two hospitals merged into one management unit in 1987. He is a member of Independent Development Council for People with Mental Handicap, a panel member of National Development Team for people with a mental handicap and Chairman of North Western Regional Advisory Group on Mental Health Services.

Professor Peter Mittler, CBE, is Professor of Special Education, University of Manchester.

James Ross has been Director of MENCAP with special responsibilities for the organisation's Welfare and Counselling Services and International Affairs. He serves on a number of Government committees and other national bodies connected with the provision of services and benefits for disabled people.

His current appointments include: Director of Tadworth Court Children's Hospital; Vice Chairman of the Voluntary Council for Handicapped Children; Board of Management of the Disability Alliance; the Children's Policy Review Group and the National Children's Bureau.

Dr Yvonne V. Wiley graduated at Queen's University, Belfast. She is currently Senior Lecturer in the Department of Mental Health, University of Bristol and Consultant to the Mental Handicap Unit, Frenchay Health Authority. She is also an active member of the Royal College of Psychiatrists and President of the Bristol branch of MENCAP.

Introduction

Alan Leighton
Consultant Group Director, Marketing and Communications,
MENCAP

The majority of people with a mental handicap have always been cared for by their parents. Like those who have been looked after in long stay institutions, they have only recently begun to be accepted as citizens within the community. And it is mainly as a result of parental pressure that their needs are beginning to be acknowledged alongside the needs of those fortunate enough to be referred to as 'normal'.

National policy now accepts that children with a mental handicap should not live in hospitals and that adults should be 'phased out' of institutional care into smaller homes. The principles and policy were first outlined in a Government White Paper, 'Better Services for the Mentally Handicapped' (1971) and since then developments have taken place to implement those proposals.

The basic principle underlying community care and outlined in the White Paper is that 'appropriate care should be provided for individuals in such a way as to enable them to lead as normal an existence as possible given their particular disabilities and to minimise disruption of life within their community'. For community care to become a reality it must encompass a whole range of services which cater for the additional and special needs of people who are mentally handicapped. It should also bring about access to the 'ordinary' services and opportunities for individuals and families which others take for granted. It also entails the task of bringing about an overall awareness of those needs and this inevitably involves, in the first instance, an acceptance of people who are mentally handicapped.

However, before real acceptance of people with a mental handicap is achieved, it is necessary to eliminate misunderstandings which exist about mental handicap. For example, it is not an illness: it is not infectious, nor is it contagious. It is the result of brain malfunction and is medically irrepairable either by drug therapy or surgery. The term 'mental handicap' is used to cover a very wide spectrum of brain malfunctions, whose effects range from mild learning difficulties at one end of the scale to profound and multiple handicaps at the other. However, people who have a mental handicap can benefit from the right kind of education and training.

There is much public confusion between mental handicap and mental illness. One of the easiest ways to aid understanding of the difference is to use the illustration of the 'normal' person who suddenly suffers accidental brain injury which is irreparable. The intellect may be damaged, there may be loss of memory, or loss of physical co-ordination or there may be an inability to retain information to mention just a few of the possible effects. This sort of permanent damage is what we call mental handicap. 'Mental illness', by contrast, is generally medically treatable by various forms of therapy and a complete recovery is possible. Anyone, including people with a mental handicap, can suffer from mental illness. Although this may be an over-simplification of the difference between the two conditions, it can eliminate some of the fears which often result from ignorance.

A survey undertaken for MENCAP (The Royal Society for Mentally Handicapped Children and Adults) and the DHSS confirms this considerable confusion about the distinction between mental handicap and mental illness. However, it also indicates that those who have personal contact with people with a mental handicap are generally much more knowledgeable and positive about their needs. Unfortunately there is still a very large section of society which has no direct contact and consequently fears of the unknown abound and long-held prejudices become firmly entrenched.

Some of the attitudes which emerged from the survey included the following:

'Mentally handicapped people are unpredictable.'

'I am not sure how to deal with mentally handicapped people.'

'I find it easier to accept a mentally handicapped child than an adult living in the community.'

'Having mentally handicapped people in my area, I would worry about my children's safety.'

'I would worry if the family next door had a mentally handicapped child/adult.'

'The general public are very prejudiced about mentally handicapped people.'

'They would need to be carefully supervised otherwise I would worry about the community suffering.'

'I would worry about house prices going down.'

'They would need to be carefully supervised for their own protection.'

'I am not sure how to deal with them.'

'I would like to know how to help them if they were living in my area.'

'It's only appropriate for those with less severe handicaps to be living in the community.'

Such attitudes can be reduced to five key factors:

1. **Supervision/Responsibility:** 'People with mental handicaps need to be supervised.'
2. **Contact:** 'I would help a person with mental handicap if I saw one.'
3. **Prejudice:** 'The general public are very prejudiced.'
4. **Effect on community:** 'My children will be threatened.'
5. **Confidence of contact:** 'I'm not sure how to deal with mentally handicapped people.'

The quantative section of the survey used the following methodology:

1 A representative sample of 450 adults aged 16+ recruited and interviewed in their own home.
2. The sample quota were controlled by age, sex, social class and area to ensure representation.
3. Interviews were conducted in 39 areas, of which 10 areas were included due to opposition encountered where attempts were made to establish a community home.
4. The questionnaire was fully piloted.
5. The field work was conducted from 3 to 10 July 1987.
6. At the analysis stage, multi–variate analysis was conducted in order to identify consumer groupings of attitudes.

The respondents' subsequent 'scores' on each of the 1 to 5 Factors were entered into a cluster analysis program and as a result four cluster groupings were identified.

Cluster 1: Avoiders (25%)

These are people who generally had less contact with people who are mentally handicapped and where contact was made it was in the street or through watching television. They are concerned about any direct contact, especially with severe handicap. They are not interested in understanding or helping in any way at all. They express their reasons as being out of concern for the community and for their family. They are the most prejudiced group but don't consider that people are prejudiced. They are anti-integration.

Cluster 2: Protectors (27%)

This group firmly believe that careful supervision would be necessary for integration. Their attitudes towards unspecific contact is similar to that of people who are sympathetic to care in the community. They express concern about the effect on the community and family and would like to be consulted if integration is to take place. They are concerned about severe cases of disability and feel that people with a mental handicap can be violent and unpredictable. They are generally in favour of integration but only with careful supervision and NOT in their own backyard.

Cluster 3: Naïve acceptors (26%)

There is a high proportion of 16–24 year olds in this group and they are very much in favour of the family taking responsibility for mentally handicapped people. They disregard the need for supervision although they do believe that people are prejudiced. They feel that people who have a mental handicap should lead a normal life and be treated as normal. They would encourage contact but don't feel confident to do so. They have no concerns for the community but are less happy to accept mentally handicapped adults. They are highly positive about integration but naïve and idealistic. This group would be most open to adverse publicity, area activists and disturbing experiences. Their attitudes are likely to change with increasing age.

Cluster 4: Confident acceptors (22%)

This is the group who are most likely to have had contact, and especially direct contact, through close friends or family. They appreciate the need for supervision particularly for the protection of people who have mental handicaps. They believe that such people are the same as everyone else and that they should be treated as such. They feel comfortable with direct contact. They have no concern about the effect on the community and would accept both children and adults. They have a highly positive approach towards integration and may become actively involved.

Summary

It would appear that the general public react quite favourably in principle to the programme of integration. However, doubts exist about the level of supervision provided in the more severe cases. Only just over half of the sample surveyed had any experience of contact with people who are mentally handicapped and there is evidence that those reacting most favourably had had the greatest direct contact. Around one quarter of the sample hold favourable benevolent attitudes and actively encourage integration, whilst a similar proportion have no interest in people with mental handicap and are therefore anti-integration.

The remaining 50% are sympathetic towards people with mental handicap but half of this group (26% overall) are rather naïve and idealistic and fail to understand potential problems. This group (many of which are 16–24 years) are less confident about dealing with mentally handicapped people and therefore their attitudes might potentially change with contact and increasing age.

The remaining 25% of the sample hold similar attitudes to the 'Acceptors' groups but would react negatively if the integration programme affected their family or community well-being. This group would need reassurance, particularly concerning supervision and responsibility, if people with mental handicap were to be integrated close by.

The awareness of existing schemes for integration was measured at a low level (17%) but the greater majority of those aware reacted favourably to the scheme. Although this survey specifically dealt with attitudes towards integration the prime objective was to provide an understanding of the general public's major prejudices towards people who are mentally handicapped.

The aim of the contributors of this book is to attempt to bring about a greater understanding and awareness of the special needs of people who have a mental handicap. These needs include opportunities for education and training, transport facilities, employment opportunities, community medical services, family support services, appropriate social security benefits, facilities for recreation and leisure but, perhaps, above all is the need for individuals to have 'choices' within all these areas. People with a mental handicap should be given every opportunity to express themselves and to be involved in the process of choice not simply as an academic exercise, but as a reality. It is our hope that the views that have been expressed will enable those who are involved in the care and support of people with a mental handicap to understand and extend the area of choice that is available.

PART ONE

The background to care in the community

CHAPTER 1

From villains to victims

Andy Alaszewski
Senior Lecturer in Health and Social Policy, University of Hull

In this short introductory chapter, the aim has not been to provide a comprehensive history of the development of attitudes towards and services for mentally handicapped people. Readers who want more detail may consult the collection of essays edited by Gabbay (1983), Ayer and Alaszewski (1986, pp. 3–68) or Alaszewski (1986, pp. 3–34). In this chapter the emphasis is on attitudes to mentally handicapped people within official policy. In the first part of the chapter it is shown how, at the beginning of the twentieth century, official attention was drawn to mentally defective people in such a way that they were seen as a serious social threat. The second part examines the development of more positive attitudes after World War II.

Mentally handicapped people as villains: the development of attitudes at the beginning of the twentieth century

Although people were referred to as fools and simpletons before the twentieth century, such people were not seen as a 'social problem' about which governments had to have clear policies. This changed with the appointment in 1904 of a Royal Commission to investigate the problem of the 'feeble-minded'. The Royal Commission's report (1908) established the mentally defective as a distinctive problem group which required special state intervention for its care and control. To understand the radical implications of the Commission and subsequent legislation, it is necessary to examine how mentally defective people came to be seen as a problem, the perception of the causes of this problem, and the solutions which were proposed.

Mentally defective people as a problem

The identification of mentally defective people as a social problem was associated with the development of universal, compulsory elementary education. In the 1870s legislation was passed in both

England and Scotland that established a system of compulsory elementary education. The system which developed in the 1880s was based on education in literacy and numeracy. Central government appointed inspectors who tested the numeracy and literacy of pupils, and elementary teachers were paid according to the results of these tests. Elementary teachers had an incentive to identify and exclude pupils who had difficulty in acquiring the necessary skills. These children were either excluded from school or placed in special classes.

In 1889 'problem' children attracted the attention of central government and a Royal Commission was appointed to consider one such group: deaf, dumb and blind children. The Commission identified an additional category of children who created difficulties: 'feeble-minded' children. The Commission recommended that feeble-minded children should be separated from other children in public elementary schools. Following this report, the Board of Education established a departmental committee to investigate the education of feeble-minded and defective children. The committee endorsed the segregation of feeble-minded and defective children from other children and the establishment of special classes for these children. In other industrial countries there were similar developments. In France, Binet was given the task of developing a method of identifying children in Parisien schools who could not adapt themselves to the curriculum. With Simon he developed a scale for measuring intelligence. This was then used as a systematic method of screening the intelligence of school children and led to the identification within the school system of a large number of mentally defective children.

Mental defect might have remained an 'educational problem', if the identification of defectives had not coincided with a moral panic about the quality of the population. The end of the nineteenth century was a period of turmoil and unrest that culminated in World War I. Internally most European countries experienced class conflict, with the rise of working class political parties and industrial trade unions influenced by socialist or marxist ideologies. Externally there was heightening competition and tension between European countries. Some sort of imperial conflict seemed inevitable at the end of the nineteenth century. Social Darwinism had become popular and it indicated that the 'fittest' state (i.e., the state with the largest and fittest population) would survive and dominate the other states. The quality of the population was seen as a crucial factor in the impending conflict. The Boer War acted as a focus for the anxieties of the ruling élite. Not only did the British Army suffer embarrassing reverses at the hands of a small group of Dutch farmers in South Africa, but a large number of the conscripts had to be rejected as medically unfit. An inter-departmental committee was established on physical deterioration and when this reported in 1904 it tended to confirm the worst fears. Mental defect changed from being an educational problem into a national problem.

The cause of national degeneracy: the inheritance of mental defect

Social Darwinism was given theoretical respectability by eugenists. A number of investigators undertook 'scientific studies' that purported to show that both intelligence and mental defect were inherited. For example, Goddard in a study of the descendents of an American Revolutionary War soldier tried to 'show that mental deficiency and more generally, its connection with crime, pauperism and prostitution was inherited according to Mendelian laws' (Ray, 1983, p.219).

Initially the views of eugenists were restricted to an intellectual minority but 'in the Edwardian era few social movements mushroomed as rapidly as did eugenics' (Barker, 1983, p.197). By 1910 eugenics had become accepted both in the press and political debates. Not only was there a fear that mental defectives were extremely fertile, but there was a belief that they did not respond to normal moral constraints and tended to produce more offspring than other people. To control what was seen as a rising threat to the quality of the race, a number of societies were established for the care and control of mental defectives and campaigned to raise public consciousness. In 1904 the government responded by appointing a Royal Commission, which reported in 1908. The eugenists had an important influence on the findings of the Commission. The Commission accepted the eugenists' arguments that mental defect was a threat to society and that it was caused by the reproduction of existing defectives who tended to have more offspring than other people.

The solution: segregation in institutions

As eugenists identified the cause of the 'mental deficiency problem' as the inheritance of undesirable characteristics, they advocated social engineering to improve the characteristics of the population. This social engineering was to take the form of positive eugenics to develop the more positive characteristics of the population, and negative eugenics to reduce the undesirable characteristics. Positive eugenics never got much beyond exhortation to the upper classes to have more children. Negative eugenics had more impact. It involved the development of strategies to prevent undesirable, especially mentally defective, people from having children. As mental defectives were not seen as responsive to normal social and moral pressures they had to be clearly identified and controlled. The 1913 Mental Deficiency Act created a special legal status for mentally defective people. Low-grade defectives were classified as imbeciles and idiots and their defect was seen as self-evident. No additional evidence was required to make these defectives suitable for care under the provisions of the Act. In contrast, high-grade defect, feeble–mindedness and moral defect were more difficult to define as they shaded into normality. Eugenists believed that it was important to identify these defectives as they were the source of future generations of defectives. The Act did so by specifying that high-grade defectives should be dealt with under the Act when their defect was associated with various forms of anti-social behaviour.

Once defectives had been identified, the cycle of degeneracy had to be broken by specific measures to supervise and control defectives and to prevent them reproducing. There were two main alternatives: sterilisation or segregation. Sterilisation raised serious ethical and practical problems. Until the twentieth century sterilisation involved radical surgery such as castration. There was a well-established model for segregation: the lunatic asylum. This asylum model was used in the mental deficiency institution or colony, which became the official response to the problem of mental deficiency.

Developing the institutional system: the inter-war years

The 1913 Mental Deficiency Act created a legal framework for the segregation of mental defectives but its implementation was delayed by World War I. Central government was preoccupied with the war effort, then reconstruction. Among Local Authorities there was little commitment to the Act. In the mid-1920s the Board of Education initiated a review of its responsibilities for the education of child defectives. In agreement with the Board of Control the terms of reference of the Wood Committee were expanded to include all defectives.

The reports of the Wood Committee were based on the same assumptions as the 1908 Royal Commission and the 1913 Mental Deficiency Act. Mental defectives were seen as a major cause of social problems and crime. The members of the Committee argued that mental defect was hereditary and that mental defectives had a high fertility. Indeed they wanted to 'prevent the racial disaster of mental deficiency' (Wood Committee, 1929, p.82). The Committee also endorsed the solution proposed before the War: segregation in institutions. Using the data collected by its investigators, the Committee argued that there were approximately 300,000 mental defectives in England and Wales and that 100,000 would require segregation. Following the reports, there was a rapid expansion of institutional facilities.

Summary

A combination of factors in the first decade of the twentieth century combined to identify mentally defective people as a major threat to society. The development of compulsory elementary education drew attention to children who could not acquire the basic skills of literacy and numeracy. The imperial and class tensions of the late nineteenth and early twentieth century created concerns about the quality of the population. The eugenists viewed mental deficiency as a cycle of degeneracy and offered a way of breaking this cycle through the segregation of mental defectives.

Mentally handicapped people as victims: the development of attitudes since World War II

A radical change has taken place in official attitudes towards mentally handicapped people since World War II, and a new pattern of services is beginning to emerge. The precise reasons for the changes were complex and were associated with changes that took place in and around the War. The racial fantasies of the Nazis and the grotesque development of institutions such as the extermination camp at Auschwitz undermined the credibility of eugenics. The consensus politics of the War reduced some of the class tensions. International tensions persisted but in a nuclear era the emphasis has shifted from quantity and quality of population to weapons technology and production.

There have been important changes in attitudes to mentally handicapped people. In the 1950s these changes could be seen tentatively in the report of the Royal Commission on the Law relating to Mental Illness and Mental Deficiency. In the 1970s with the publication of the White Paper *Better Services for the Mentally Handicapped* (1971) and the *Jay Report* (1979), the changes were more radical. In these official documents it is possible to identify a new problem: the institutions; a new explanation for the problem: labelling theory; and a new solution: community care.

The new problem: the institutions

After World War II, institutions came to be seen as part of the problem. In 1951 the National Council for Civil Liberties in its pamphlet *50,000 Outside the Law*, argued that institutions deprived individuals of their liberty and created the very problems that they were supposed to solve. Mentally defective people were not innately morally defective, but the institution created deviant and criminal behaviour (NCCL, 1951, front page).

A number of writers identified the debilitating and damaging effects on residents of different types of institutions. Lady Allen of Hurtwood, a distinguished voluntary worker, exposed the unimaginative and depersonalising conditions in children's homes (Allen of Hurtwood, 1945). Russell Barton, a psychiatrist, wrote a training manual for nurses in which he argued that many of the patients in the long-stay wards in British mental hospitals suffered from two diseases: an illness that was related to their admission, and a second one that was created by their stay in hospital. Goffman (1961), an American sociologist, argued, in a widely read book, that the problems were not limited to one specific type of institution but were characteristic of all institutions.

The view that institutions were the problem has now become accepted within official publications. The authors of the 1971 White Paper were preoccupied with the problems of mental handicap hospitals. They accepted the findings, and built upon the work, of academic critics by acknowledging that large-scale institutions were intrinsically dehumanising and depersonalising:

> 'In the worst places, [institutional care] produces boredom and tension and even occasional violence. Patients become apathetic and institutionalised and sink into a state of complete physical and social dependence. Nurses are frustrated by having no time to provide more than attention to basic physical needs, without using psychiatric nursing skills in which they have been trained.' (DHSS, 1971, para. 114.)

The cause of the problem: segregation and labelling

The 1913 legislation was based on the assumption that mental deficiency could easily be identified by experts, who were trained in the correct procedures. In the 1950s and 1960s sociologists began to challenge this view. They argued that the defect was not an intrinsic characteristic of the defective person but rather was created by a society's reaction to that person. Rather than asking how much mental defect existed, researchers asked how, and in what circumstance, did a person become defined as a defective. By rephrasing the problem, the centre of interest shifted from 'the victim' and his or her characteristics, to the agency which defined specific problems, gave these problems names or labels, and prescribed certain actions in response to these problems. These agencies were seen as playing an active part in the way social problems were defined and therefore created.

Dexter examined the politics of 'stupidity' and argued that mentally handicapped people suffered especially badly from society's reaction:

> 'There is . . . the experience which may be observed over and over again of the denial of employment, of legal rights, of a fair hearing, of an opportunity, to the stupid, because they are stupid (e.g. have a low IQ or show poor academic performance) and not because the stupidity is relevant to the task or claim, or situation.' (Dexter, 1964, p.4).

Researchers argued that institutions were an essential part of society's reaction to mentally handicapped people. By segregating mentally handicapped people from the rest of society, they both created and reinforced the differences between 'normal' and 'abnormal' people.

In California, Mercer researched the ways in which state schools identified and labelled people as mentally retarded. She found that although the behaviour and skills of the children played a part in the process of labelling, an equally important element in the labelling was the child's social status. Children with the same skills but different social backgrounds could be labelled and treated in very different ways. The closer a child's background was to the dominant white, Anglo-Saxon, Protestant culture, the less chance that the child would be labelled mentally retarded. Mercer argued that existing procedures, in particular IQ tests, discriminated against minority groups.

One sign of official concern about the impact of labelling on mentally handicapped people has been a rapid change of terminology. Since World War II mentally handicapped people have been referred to as mentally subnormal people, mentally handicapped people, people with learning difficulties and people with an intellectual impairment. This concern has resulted in a reluctance to use any system of classification and an emphasis on individual needs. (See, for example, *Jay Report*, 1979, and *Warnock Report*, 1978.)

Within this changing terminology, there has been a significant shift of emphasis. The eugenists were mainly interested in mildly handicapped people. They felt that these people were the major threat and required special measures to identify and to control them. There is now more emphasis on severely and profoundly handicapped people. In their case, the handicaps are so severe that there can be little doubt and little dispute about the individual's dependency and need for services and social support. In the case of mildly handicapped people, there is considerable room for such doubt.

The Royal Commission on Law Relating to Mental Illness and Mental Deficiency (1957) recommended that the whole area of mental disorder, including mental deficiency, should be reclassified. The terminology introduced by the Mental Deficiency Act should be replaced by three new categories: subnormality, severe subnormality and psychopathy. The introduction of the concept and category of psychopathy was particularly important for mentally handicapped people. It enabled much of the taint of moral defect, personality disorder and criminality, which had been associated with mental defect, to be syphoned off into this new category. The psychopaths became the 'evil' villains, whereas mentally handicapped people could be increasingly seen as innocent victims of circumstances for which they were not responsible.

The new solution: community care

If institutions have come to be the problem, then the solution is community care: shutting institutions and integrating mentally handicapped people into the community. The concept of community care can be traced back to the Royal Commission (1957). The Commission recommended, not the closure of institutions, but the development of parallel services for mentally handicapped people within local authorities. The Commission did not recommend any particular balance between institutional provision within the NHS and community provision within local authorities.

The 1971 White Paper found that, despite the recommendations of the 1957 Royal Commission and specific directions by Ministers of Health to local authorities to develop community facilities, very little progress had been made in developing community services. At the end of 1969, only 39 of the 157 local authorities in England and only four of the 70 Welsh authorities had residential provision for children and adults. The White Paper set targets to be achieved by 1991. Community residential provision was to expand from some 6,000 places to over 35,000 places. Institutional provision was to be halved with an immediate and rigorous ban on the construction or expansion of any hospital over 500 beds and an overall reduction of beds in mental handicap hospitals from 60,000 to 30,000. These hospitals were to provide services for mentally handicapped people who required medical and nursing care.

The development of official attitudes has been influenced by an explicit ideology: normalisation. In the United States, the concept has been developed by Wolfensberger (1972) and is associated with the work of the Eastern Nebraska Office of Retardation (Thomas, Firth and Kendall, 1978). In England the concept of normalisation was associated with the Campaign for Mentally Handicapped People. Advocates of normalisation argued that instead of being segregated in institutions, mentally handicapped people should have the right to experience normal life and to be integrated within the community.

The ideas of normalisation influenced the Jay Committee on mental handicap nursing and care (1979). Previous committees had tended to recommend incremental adjustments to the existing pattern of services. The Jay Committee did not start from the existing pattern of services; rather it tried to define an ideal pattern of services and to identify the elements of this ideal service. The Committee started from a philosophy of care for mentally handicapped people. The Committee made explicit the three principles that underlay this philosophy, as follows:

1. Mentally handicapped people have a right to enjoy normal patterns of life within the community.

2.   Mentally handicapped people have a right to be treated as individuals.
3.   Mentally handicapped people will require additional help from the communities in which they live and the professional services if they are to develop to their maximum potential as individuals. (Jay Committee, 1979, para. 89.)

Like the Edwardian eugenists, the Jay Committee used legal rhetoric, but whereas the eugenists used this rhetoric to deprive mentally deficient people of their rights, the Jay Committee wanted to use it to protect and enhance the rights of mentally handicapped people.

From ideology to practice: developing community care

The last thirty years have marked a radical change in official attitudes to mentally handicapped people. The positive benefits of these changes should not be underestimated. However, there are problems. Overall progress has been slow even in terms of the conservative targets of the 1971 White Paper. Institutional provision for adults should decline by over 1,100 places a year and community residential provision should increase at a marginally faster rate. Although community facilities are expanding by nearly 950 places a year institutional facilities are falling by only 640 places. In 1984 there was a short fall of 11,000 community places and an excess of 7,300 institutional places (data calculated from Audit Commission, 1986).

Although the attitudes implicit in the institutional system were negative, mentally handicapped people were the centre of official interest. Since World War II, the centre of official interest has tended to shift to the institutions and their problems. Closing institutions is presented as the means of achieving a better service for mentally handicapped people but it is too easy for the means to become the end. (See, for example, Korman and Glennerster, 1985, and the Social Services Committee, 1985).

The concept of community care is vague. It may be very useful as political rhetoric and as a symbol of changed attitudes to mentally handicapped people, but as a specific guide to service development it is useless. In the institutional system one agency took the lead in developing services. Community care means that responsibility is shared between a number of agencies. As the Audit Commission (1986) points out, progress is very patchy and 'the care that people receive is as much dependent on where they live as on what they need'.

If agencies shared a common view of the needs of mentally handicapped people, they could work together to develop an integrated package of services for mentally handicapped people and their families. There is little evidence that integrated services are developing. As mentally handicapped people grow older, they are passed from agency to agency. Young children's main contact is with the doctors, health visitors and clinical psychologists of the health service. During school years their main contact is with teachers and educational psychologists. As they get older they have increasing contact with social workers and community mental handicap nurses. The variety of professionals can be confusing, their expertise and attitudes extremely different, and their co-ordination poor.

Conclusion

Through an unfortunate combination of circumstances mentally deficient people became the focus of official interest at the beginning of this century. They were seen as a major threat to society that could be controlled through the development of an institutional system. Although official interest shifted to other social problems, the institutional system expanded under its own dynamics reaching a peak of 60,000 beds at the end of the 1960s.

When mentally handicapped people again attracted widespread attention, it was through the short-comings of the institutions. The institutions are now the problem rather than the solution and mentally handicapped people are the victims of past attitudes and inappropriate services.

Further reading

1. Alaszewski, A., *Institutional Care and the Mentally Handicapped: The Mental Handicap Hospital* (Croom Helm, 1986).
2. Allen of Hurtwood, Lady, *Whose Children?* (Simkin Marshall, 1945).
3. Audit Commission, *Making a Reality of Community Care* (HMSO, 1986).
4. Ayer, S., Alaszewski, A., *Community Care and the Mentally Handicapped: Services for Mothers and their Mentally Handicapped Children* (Croom Helm, 1986).
5. Barker, D., 'How to Curb the Fertility of the Unfit: the Feeble-minded in Edwardian Britain', *Oxford Review of Education*, vol. 9 (1983), pp. 197–211.
6. Barton, R., *Institutional Neurosis* (John Wright, Bristol, 1959).
7. Dexter, L. A., 'On the Politics and Sociology of Stupidity in our Society', H. S. Becker (ed), *The Other Side: Perspectives on Deviance* (The Free Press, New York, 1964).
8. DHSS, *Better Services for the Mentally Handicapped* (Cmnd. 4683, HMSO, 1971).
9. Gabbay, J., (ed), 'Mental Handicap and Education', *Oxford Review of Education*, vol. 9 (1983), Special Issue.
10. Goffman, E., *Asylums* (Doubledays, New York, 1961).

11. Jay Committee, *Report of the Committee of Enquiry into Mental Handicap Nursing and Care, Vol 1* (Cmnd. 7468–I, HMSO, 1979).
12. Korman, N., Glennerster, H., *Closing a Hospital: The Darenth Park Project* (Bedford Square Press, 1985).
13. Mercer, J. R., *Labeling the Mentally Retarded*, (University of California Press, California, 1973).
14. Ray, L. J., 'Eugenics, Mental Deficiency and Fabian Socialism between the Wars', *Oxford Review of Education*, vol. 9 (1983), pp. 213–22.
15. Royal Commission, *Report of The Royal Commission on the Care and Control of the Feeble-Minded* (Cmnd. 4202, HMSO, 1908).
16. Royal Commission, *Report of the Royal Commission on the Law Relating to Mental Illness and Mental Deficiency, 1954–1957* (Cmnd., 169, HMSO, 1957).
17. Social Services Committee, *Second Report, Session 1984–1985, Community Care* (Chairman, Renee Short), (HC, 13–I, HMSO, 1985).
18. Thomas, D., Firth, H., Kendall, A., *ENCOR – A Way Ahead* (Campaign for Mentally Handicapped People, 1978).
19. Wolfensberger, W., *The Principle of Normalization in Human Services* (Leonard Crainford, Toronto, 1972).
20. Warnock Report, *Special Educational Needs: Report of the Committee of Enquiry into the Education of Handicapped Children and Young People* (Cmnd. 7212, HMSO, 1978).
21. Wood Committee, *Report of the Mental Deficiency Committee, Part III, The Adult Defective* (HMSO, 1929).

CHAPTER 2

Closing the hospitals and changing provision

Tom McLean, MBE
Director of Nursing Services, Calderstones

It is sometimes forgotten that the contraction of hospital services for people with mental handicap in England and Wales has been in train for many years. Since the initial exodus of people following the passage of the 1959 Mental Health Act, the reduction has been more a result of deaths and changes in admission patterns and length of stay than of any concerted effort to rehabilitate people who might need any more than minimal support. Thought about relocating the more dependant people from hospital to care in communities has evolved from very general and hazy ideas based on the undesirability of the large-scale, single-campus institutions rather than from any clear concept of meeting individual needs.

Concern about the maximum size of hospitals being not more than 500 places, and later not more than 200, seem now to have ignored the fact that the largest, potentially most unattractive, place is composed of sub-units of no greater size than the average hostel or the units found in smaller hospitals. It should not be forgotten that some of the worst scandals of the 1960s and 1970s occurred in smaller hospitals. In short, the purpose-built non-campus units are really no smaller, often no better, than average wards in many of our large hospitals. However, this has only been recently realised.

Until the recent emphasis on a truly individual focus of attention for people with mental handicap, an essential component of thinking was the concept of the locally-based hospital unit developed in the Wessex region in the 1970s. These units offered severely and multiply handicapped adults residential care of the kind which hostels already provided for those who were mildly handicapped and for children, and represented the first major shift from the large campus provision for this group. Ministry of Health statements about minimum standards had already stimulated this theme in 1964, choosing as indicators areas of living and sleeping space, of personal storage space, and privacy within the targets of reduced ward size. These standards in themselves did little to alter the fact that people continued to live in public or to give any possibility of real freedom of choice for the individuals concerned.

The desirable improvements in the physical environment which followed Richard Crossman's initiatives of the late 1960s – prefabricated 24-bed units and more money for improvements to existing stock – turned out to be no more than experiences in domestication, so easily confused with a truly domestic outcome. This criticism may be summarised as the difference between home and home-like, a phrase often used in describing what we felt mentally handicapped people needed, to be found, for example, in the principles laid down in the 1971 White Paper *Better Services for the Mentally Handicapped.*

The rolls of wallpaper which covered up the green paint of former generations certainly made for a more pleasant appearance but did this really make a ward into a home? How could cosmetic exercises of this kind do more than salve the conscience of society and hospital managers whilst hiding the real truth? Truths about the denials of freedom of choice; about the failure to develop skills, friendships, self-confidence or self-respect for the vast majority of people who were admitted. None of the DHSS indicators used asked what was happening to people or sought to find out what it felt like to be on the receiving end.

A major confusion in residential services, cause of debate and some trouble, is the lack of clarity between everyday living experience and a quite separate notion of treatment. It is now realised that long-term treatment, which divorces people from the opportunity to continue to practice and develop the skills of everyday life, cannot succeed.

The difficulty which people with handicaps have in generalising experience from artificial training situations into everyday life on discharge from hospitals often leads to failure and re-admission after an apparently successful outcome as judged by performance in the hospital regime. A structured approach which maintains or develops personal, social and everyday living skills must remain a major component in meeting the needs of individuals, and in successfully modifying undesirable behaviour. Participation in all aspects of life with necessary staff support is, in itself, often a treatment.

It is obvious that the provision of centrally-organised support services such as domestic services, catering and supplies departments can work against a completely personalised programme approach of this nature unless there is a clear agreement between clinical and service departments.

Any insistence that regular involvement in, for example, shopping and cooking is necessary to meet individual needs can cause difficulty with these departments. When the problems arising from these clashes of interest are resolved by the provision of artificial training opportunities totally unrelated to normal rhythms and taking place outside the home unit, they meet only the needs of staff groups seeking to prevent upset within the organisation. It is hardly surprising, given the scale of operation, that these services should have been arranged in a centralised way. But even now where there is recognition of the value of participation in all aspects of daily living as a part of treatment, it is almost impossible to permit this life-style in the institutional model.

Even in special training areas in hospitals and in Adult Training Centres because of the scale of the operation and needs of the majority, we often see the exclusion of a person with problem behaviour until, it is said, such time as their behaviour improves. This leaves people inactive in the ward, lengthens the time taken to effect the 'cure', a situation often further aggravated by a reluctance to accept people back because of their history and reputation.

If, in the future, this state of affairs is not to be repeated, a major challenge to community services will be the creation of a non-buck-passing attitude in staff. This might be assisted by the development of responsive local specialist teams designed to give extra support to people where they live. The alternative strategy of moving people to special units where they are congregated together with others having the same difficulties will simply perpetuate the problems of former times.

Towards greater independence

Persuading staff to appreciate the relevance of client participation in everyday activity on a regular basis, even where it would be quicker or more efficient for staff to do the work themselves, is, surprisingly, still necessary. In spite of research showing that resident-staff interaction is limited to about ten minutes a day we still see staff carrying out simple house-keeping tasks alone whilst residents sit indulging in self-stimulating activity.

The recent introduction of the Individual Programme Plans (IPP), a system involving staff groups concerned in assessment of individuals and planning, delivering and maintaining programmes has focused attention on individual needs and the best way of meeting them. Thorough discussions of the service deficiency reports, which are an integral part of the system, have also helped managers to clarify some of the dilemmas which highlight the friction between individual needs and organisational needs and to question some restrictive practices.

IPP is a technique which helps staff recognise the artificiality of the divide between patterns of ordinary daily life and treatment. There is little point in pursuing the IPP approach without the participation, at each and every opportunity, of the residents themselves, their families or advocates, and, as we move towards the resettlement of hospital residents, staff from receiving districts also.

Emerging policy on the model of care which helps resolve some of the problems by allowing people to participate in everyday life involves the use of ordinary housing. The Jay Committee model of residential care, endorsed now by many authorities and elaborated upon by the Kings' Fund Ordinary Life initiative, was given the Government's seal of approval in the 1982 statement *Care in Action* 'for all but a very small minority'.

Real homes are gradually being established in many parts of the country: most encouraging projects have been described in, for example, Leeds, Trafford, Camden, Northumberland, Wessex, Lancashire and Bristol and new developments are rapidly increasing. Attempts to change the standard of care for people with additional special needs by the adoption of the ordinary life model have often been thwarted by a lack of back-up, knowledge, expertise or confidence to deal with multiple handicaps and behaviour problems. Thus we see a demand for special units for some people, rather than the development of real support mechanisms to enable those with additional problems to remain in the community. Meeting the needs of people with challenging behaviours by the provision of special units only perpetuates the spiral of deprivation. We have these units now: they are called hospitals. There seems to be little point in wasting capital to provide more of these when we might attempt to develop the alternative model of support teams. This suggestion has the advantage of trial without a fifty-year commitment to bricks and mortar.

The understandable pleasure at improving any environment in the way in which we have over the past few years should not be seen as the end of the matter. If we are not to be told by visiting members of parliament that our hospitals are now 'better than my boarding school' (Conservative) or are 'not as bad as national service' (Labour) we must continue to recognise the short-comings of the approach which does no more than to tart-up what went before rather than establishing any new opportunities. Local training workshops on normalisation involving not only care workers but planners seem essential if these confusions are to be eliminated. Even where programmes of modernisation are carried out, so powerful are the former models of mass treatment, so incomplete our grasp of normalisation and so ingrained our double standards that former practices remain unless there is a continuing investment in staff training.

Unless we constantly acknowledge how awful the quality of life is in even the smartest of modernised facilities we shall be seduced by the superficial into thinking that fifteen, or ten, or five in a dormitory is good enough provided the wallpaper is nice.

Improving the physical environment has been a major preoccupation without any real examination of what goes on within the newly created, often smaller, places. Albert Kushlick's work on measurement of 'engagement' led to a heightened awareness of the real extent of the empty hours in the 1970s. The extent to which outings, even to a local shop, and contact with non-handicapped people other than paid staff are still, at worst, treats, or at best weekly occurrences rather than everyday experiences. For such experiences to assist in treatment or individual development there must be an ability on the part of the student if not to actually remember the last such event, then for experiences to be frequent enough to be useful cumulatively.

Closing hospitals and moving resources

Against a background of gradual change in the expectations of families, the hospital scandals, the development of alternative models of thinking, decision-making about hospital closure has been an equally gradual and un-co-ordinated process, driven, it seems, by factors only secondarily connected to the needs of individuals, such as the appalling state of the buildings.

At a time of financial stringency, the policy is used only to switch resources to care in the community without any real injection of new money. The Green Paper *Care in the Community* (1981), a consultative document on moving resources for care in England, was based on the simple assumption that the combined costs of hostel accommodation and an ATC place were less than the average cost of a hospital place and this seemed justification in itself to switch funding from hospital to community. The Green Paper offered seven options for consideration. The consultation period resulted in the publication of *Health Circular (83)6, Local Authority Circular (83)5* which permitted the transfer of hospital resources to the community and set up a number of pilot projects.

Regional plans have, for some time, reflected this policy in terms of reducing hospital places in line with the development of local services. The arrival, in 1983, of the NHS annual ministerial review process switched the emphasis from one of hospital contraction to one of closure in the North Western Region and with greater emphasis on contraction targets in other parts of the country. This emphasis is all very well provided that it does result in the provision of local service and not an empty-at-all-costs mentality with little thought about the quality of that which replaces hospitals. There is a great danger that because the cash-flow generated by the contraction programme is insufficient on a per capita basis that there will be a net reduction in the total number of places provided in the new service. In this connection it must not be forgotten that the costs in hospitals also include the training budget for RNMH nurses and that, unless specifically safeguarded, this will be handed out piecemeal as places are transferred and disappear as an identifiable training resource.

Preparation of people for relocation is an extremely complex matter which includes Individual Programme Planning involving the handicapped person, relatives, staff of hospitals and receiving agencies. Selection for inclusion in plans is followed by detailed assessment, consideration of friendship patterns and design of programmes for preparation. Much emphasis has been placed upon the need for good preparation and training for resettlement in the community. However, experience in both hospitals and receiving districts shows that hospital assessment is optimistic, levels of support needed are under-estimated and predictions about possible reductions of support after an initial period of adjustment are not fulfilled. But one major, proven use of pre-resettlement grouping and preparation has been the testing of compatibilities within groups of people before discharge.

Hospital services have improved in quality in the past few years as admission patterns have shifted towards short stays for respite care or treatment, gradually replacing long-stay patterns and releasing some resources. Until recently these resources have remained in hospital. The huge increase in staffing – double in ten years – as the resident population has dramatically decreased underlines the abysmal levels of service given in the past and does not reflect in the slightest the level of investment which would be necessary to deliver service of even a reasonable standard in this model. Savings are now being used up as people are resettled, so as the under-funded are funding the unfunded there is a distinct danger that quality will suffer for those who remain in hospitals.

Hospitals have never, even at the height of their glory, provided for all people with mental handicap. There have always been waiting lists. Inability to provide for everyone does not seem adequate justification for doing nothing within the resources available. It is as well that the recent Audit Commission Report has corrected one impression surrounding current policy, which suggests that if all the cash in hospitals were transferred to care in the community, all would be well, without promise of new money.

Although it is true that hospital contraction which falls short of closure will leave us with more expensive hospitals it seems inevitable that the availability of alternative services for people with additional problems will take some time to establish. Discharges to the community into a worthwhile model of care which will enhance quality of life, rather than shift people from one institution to another, will cost more.

The phrase 'rush to the community' which put, alongside Mrs

Short's famous slogan, 'any fool can close a hospital', combined with the very high profile publicity excited by Rescare (the National Society for Mentally Handicapped People in Residential Care) gives an impression of hordes descending upon an unwelcoming public. This notion really does need to be kept in perspective.

In her excellent study of hospital closures in the 1980s, Alison Werthiemer points out what is really happening. Her results point to neither a shift of resources nor of people to real community alternatives. Of 539 people affected by hospital closure in her study over 85% transferred to other hospitals, NHS community units or local authority hostels. In the North Western Region where contraction is given high priority the total resettled between 1984 and 1986 was 360: this in a population of 4.3 million divided between 19 health districts and Liverpool in the neighbouring Mersey Region. Hardly the swamping which is claimed. However, it is a fact that where discharges have been proceeding at a reasonable rate, to Bolton for example, where efforts have been made to include people with handicaps in mainstream adult education services by the provision of tutors for that purpose, some of the classes are in danger of becoming mainly mental handicap groupings. Some family practitioners have expressed a fear that they will be swamped numerically or unable to cope with referrals made for people with special needs such as challenging behaviour or severe epilepsy. In Lancashire the Family Practitioner Committee has funded the appointment of an officer for a two-year programme of education for the GPs and to quantify the real extent of the work load caused by the hospital closure programme.

Moving into the community: planning and problems

As well as good individual programme planning for each person to be relocated, each project for the relocation of a group of people from hospital needs careful planning by all concerned. A house or number of houses in a scheme will need a project team which includes the people with handicaps themselves, staff who know residents well, representatives of families, and staff from the receiving district services. This arrangement has been most successful in resolving the problems which occur in relation to social security benefits, family fears about support levels, risk-taking and similar questions about just how the scheme would work for a particular person or group.

After responsibility is transferred to the receiving district the involvement of the hospital staff who are not actually transferring will gradually decrease. It is essential, however, that a support group for each house or cluster of houses continues to meet even when all is going well: this is vital to problem-solving, the continued motivation and morale of staff, the maintenance of standards and the development of new ideas.

Staff training and renewal, much easier to organise in larger settings, must be included in all schemes. Where staff are supporting people in smaller, dispersed settings this becomes of paramount importance. The difficulties of arranging for release of staff must be faced or plans must develop to include peripatetic officers or teams to train the staff to meet their specific needs.

In some areas there are allegations of neglect of people discharged from hospitals and who are assessed as requiring only intermittent staff intervention. This is a particularly difficult area needing great skill on the part of visiting staff. Often pointed out as failures of resettlement, people in this group will reject help when all is going well and refuse to attend traditional day activities. The field social-work approach is frequently not directional enough when compared with the nursing regime from which the person has been released. Community support workers and their trainers need to bear this in mind when schemes are set up. Margaret Flynn's research ('A study of prediction in the community placements of adults who are mentally handicapped, 1983 to 1986', University of Manchester, 1986) has some pertinent lessons about this group of people.

Much debate has taken place in the past few years about the model of residential care which is best suited to meet the needs of people with mental handicap. Until the Jay Committee expounded principles underpinning the smaller scale provision we had not seen the universal promulgation of explicit statements of principles about people and their place in the community or about service design. Following the Jay Committee the Guys Plan was published and the Kings' Fund Ordinary Life group produced their work. The adoption of this work by many authorities and agencies has produced considerable debate often leading to resistance on behalf of parents, nursing staff and psychiatrists. The feelings expressed are often combined with anxiety about the unlikelihood of staff being able to succeed where they, to quote many parents, have themselves failed. This argument overlooks the fact that the comparison is being made between on the one hand a family (or perhaps more accurately a mother) giving 24-hour care with, on the other, a rota system involving several staff, each one of whom arrives refreshed to do one shift of duty before leaving.

If the main advantages of the ordinary life model are to do with meeting the needs of individuals, with quality, integration, reduction of stigma, opportunity to learn and develop, then the other side of the coin is about the difficulty of achieving quality and about protecting the public, meeting the needs of families and not disrupting an already established regime. Families of people who are presently in the parental home add to these views in expressing the fear that resources available to them will be reduced in the situation, as they see it, of discharged people absorbing more than their fair share: often known as the 'two tier' service.

Parents often express anxiety about change to what they see as an untested system. They quite overlook the fact that most people with mental handicap live in the community in ordinary housing following normal patterns of life. Families have also argued that space is a major issue in the lives of people with mental handicap. They have perhaps fallen victim to myths about the ordinary housing model of residential care: all hospital residents are not being discharged to small council houses with many near neighbours. The wide range of ordinary housing being used includes many different sizes, some with larger than average gardens, and some on the edge of communities where a noisy and restless person could live without causing significant disruption.

Risks connected with going out of doors unescorted are often cited without too much discussion. Undeniably there is a small number of people who presently fall between those in the group who can leave hospital unescorted, use public transport and return safely, and those who cannot even leave the wards to move about the campus of the hospital without assistance. Most of the people in this middle group are amenable to training and the much better ratios of staff to residents to be found in community settings in the ordinary life model can be utilised in ways not previously possible. The experiences of hospital residents and staff who holiday together in small groups also point to what is possible. Protection without any opportunity to even a degree of independence is degrading and restricts development.

The small scale of living in the proposed neighbourhood schemes makes use of volunteers a real possibility. The employment of part-time staff for quite short spans of duty timed to meet individual mobility or escort needs becomes a worthwhile proposition, given that for local applicants this does not involve lengthy or costly travel to work. Such an arrangement also has the advantage of involving more local people in the service.

There is no doubt that failures in community care will occur. It will be for managers, agencies, staff organisations and watchdog bodies to face these honestly and ask what it will take to prevent or reduce recurrence rather than to declare the whole system a failure. It is as foolish to talk only of the failures of community care as it would be to talk only of the successes of the hospital system. To do so is to deny the very life-style which we value for ourselves and to ignore the lessons of hospital scandals and the evidence of our own eyes.

Responsibility for residential services

The contraction of hospitals leads, inevitably, to an examination of the notion of single-agency responsibility for residential services.

This is the central issue, the main argument, the outstandingly important power struggle. Arguments about domiciliary team work, about day services, about superimposed mental illness, about access to health professionals, about joint planning or any other matter are entirely peripheral. This single issue carries with it not only the major portion of resources but the undeniable major input into the lives of the clients, the major influence upon the individual, and the power base to influence all other potential influences.

The recent Commons Social Services Select Committee Report and the Audit Commission Report both follow the logic and inevitability of present trends and practice which point to a future social services leadership role. This notion draws strength from the obvious inappropriateness of ill-health as an image for the client group, leading as it does to expectations of dependence and a dependency role for the recipients of care.

Arguments between the social model and nursing take up enormous amounts of energy in defending the positions of social work staff and nurses. Exaggerations about the present ability of social service departments to provide, with appropriate health support (this phrase usually undefined), a comprehensive service are challenged by generalised woolly statements about those needing medical and nursing care (this usually undefined).

It is true that many social services departments do not have sufficient, experienced, trained staff at the present time to meet the needs of all people with mental handicap; neither do they have middle management or specialist workers to effectively support, supervise and improve practice. Many have not recognised a need to review existing practice within their own areas of responsibility: whilst joining in the debate about the undesirability of institutional care in hospitals, they perpetuate institutional models in the community.

If social services are to be the major providers for the future, then the importance of the transitional phase to the success of that future must be recognised, debated and planned. Changes in the recent past within health services must be recognised and built upon; to ignore them will be to set back the base line for future development rather than spring forward from the success. In the successful development of ordinary life residential supports for people with severe and profound mental handicap – including some with behaviour disorders – the health service nursing-led projects by far outstrip the other agencies.

It must also be recognised that basic training for the RNMH, notwithstanding the unsuitability of a medical model, has improved beyond all recognition. The syllabus and practice and training in community settings is producing a firm basis for specialist workers with knowledge, skills, experience, confidence and commitment which cannot be abandoned, either deliberately by edict on the future shape of service, or insidiously by gradual service changes. To do so without replacing these specialists with workers equally well-prepared to do the multiplicity of specialist tasks in residential and day activity support, behavioural work, service management and leadership would be irresponsible.

At the present time these are approaching 3,000 RNMH nurses in training against the small proportion of the 450 Certificate in Social Services (CSS) students who are taking a mental handicap specialist option. Added to this is the fact that the financial resources for training nurses are included in the transfer of cash from hospital to community. There is no evidence that any of this is being set on one side for basic training in the future. It is the opinion of some nurses that health authorities are not only colluding in the demise of community-based specialist training (RNMH) but appear unconcerned about what is to stand in its place. The statutory obligation placed upon health authorities to monitor expenditure when resources are transferred should include arrangements for safeguarding a specialist training for the future. It does not appear that this is being done. It will be so easy to assign responsibility retrospectively for the demise of a cohort of trained staff, but such wisdom will not fill the gap after the event.

The staff problems arising from the switch to community care derive not only from the conditions of service issues, although these are important (in particular the optional retirement, at 55, of mental health officers) but also from the much deeper cultural differences inherent in their training. Examples of success in provision of community mental handicap teams do not answer this entirely, though the differences can be successfully exploited to produce a balanced CMHT. Responsibility for the quality of professional work is contingent upon retaining control of the resources utilised to support people with mental handicap. In this respect social services staff see nurses as too controlling and directive and in turn nurses feel that social services staff are non-directive even on occasions where this is essential, for example, in dealing with behaviour problems, skill training, supporting severely handicapped people and those who do not understand the outcomes of choices made, or who have previously been deeply affected by former restrictive regimes.

These differences are only too clearly demonstrated by the continued referral of certain people to the care of nurses in hospitals because of a lack of locally-available resources and the inability of present staff to cope. The pattern, frequency and overall number of admissions could be dramatically reduced by a recognition of the need for health authorities to pursue the establishment of local, ordinary life residential services. These services would be much more successful if in an interim period of about ten years leading up to a natural, desirable, logical handover to social services, nurses be permitted to transfer to the community and continue to practice as nurses. Such projects will be successful because staff will be better managed by experienced nurses; they will have more confidence in a transfer to community work within the agency profession known to them.

The often-used argument against what is pejoratively called parallel development really is specious in the neighbourhood model because the amount of service developed is precisely that needed. Equally the quantity of middle-management support developed is exactly the amount demanded. The wasteful prospect of a facility in each agency pursuing the same client group with offers of 'a bed' cannot occur in a needs-led ordinary life residential service.

A way must be found to enable this transition to be sensibly worked out.

Remaining hospital residents

In the preoccupation with changing the location of hospital residents we must not forget the quality of service for the people who remain in hospitals, perhaps for ten or fifteen years. There is now a body of knowledge about the components of good services in the community, and as we gain experience we shall get better at providing these. At the same time, people in hospital have the right to good day services, and a standard of residential care which is not worsened by the adverse effects of the contraction plans. Bridging finance, good planning and the retention of some high-quality qualified staff within the hospital service is essential if the scandals of the 1970s are not to be repeated.

CHAPTER 3

The law and mental handicap

M. J. Gunn
Lecturer in Law, University of Nottingham

The encouragement of the community care option for people with mental handicaps has contributed to an increased interest in, and concern with, the law as it affects such people. It is asserted that one of the functions of the law is to value people as individuals and as members of society. The valuing process does not demand that people, who are in some way disadvantaged, simply be left to their own devices. The United Nations Declaration on the Rights of Mentally Retarded Persons (1971) makes this point in article 1:

'The mentally retarded person has, to the maximum degree of feasibility, the same rights as other human beings.'

Valuing people as individuals and members of society demands that the law achieves a proper balance between facilitating an independent life-style involving personal decision-making and the need to protect people with mental handicaps from exploitation and abuse. This balance expects that people with mental handicaps have as much independence of action and decision as possible, but that decisions should be taken on behalf of, and for the benefit of, a person with a mental handicap when s/he is incapable of securing them for him/herself.

The law, therefore, needs to be flexible and effective in response to satisfy these demands, which means that the law must take into account the capacities of each individual who has a mental handicap. If s/he is incapable, then there must be a means of overcoming that incapacity for the benefit of the individual. The question, therefore, is whether English law does achieve this balance and fulfil these demands. This is considered by looking at a number of legal issues of real concern for people with mental handicaps.

Management of property and affairs

At first sight the legal mechanism for managing and administering a person's property and affairs (Re: W(EEM), 1971, Chancery

Reports 123) within the Mental Health Act 1983 (Part VII, sections 93–113) does seem to be satisfactory. The Act does not presume that a person is incapable simply because s/he has a 'mental disorder'. Rather it indicates that steps can be taken only if it is decided by a judge that the individual in question is 'incapable of managing and administering his property and affairs by reason of mental disorder . . .'. 'Mental disorder' is defined sufficiently widely to cover all people who have a mental handicap. (See section 1, MHA, and Spencer, D. A., (letter) and Gunn, M. J., (reply) in *Mental Handicap*, vol II (1983), p.174).

The judge, therefore, decides whether the particular individual is capable of looking after money and property, and cannot assume that because a person has a mental handicap that s/he is incapable of taking the relevant types of decisions. What, then, does capacity mean? It would seem proper to suggest that capacity does not mean the taking of consistently correct decisions, otherwise most people would be thought to be incapable! Capacity in property issues would appear to require the ability to work out what a person has, what needs to be done with it (how money should be spent or saved and how property should be looked after), what the possible options are to achieve the desired ends and how to choose between them.

The law, therefore, is flexible in responding to the individual's capacities, but this is only part of the issue. The means by which the law deals with the property of the incapable person has been open to considerable criticism. The only general way of dealing with another's property and affairs is through the Court of Protection, although with regard to the specific case of welfare benefits, a person can be appointed by the DHSS to receive and spend them on behalf of an incapable recipient. Court of Protection receivers are appointed wherever possible. The person appointed is usually a relative of the incapable person. S/he is given the power to take many decisions in relation to the property and affairs of an incapable person. The Court retains overall jurisdiction and is unlikely to allow a receiver to spend large sums of money. If a new house needs to be purchased or the existing house needs to be altered, the receiver will need to obtain the permission of the Court before the work can go ahead and be paid for, even if there is more than enough money in the 'patient's' account to cover the cost. The receiver will not be able to write a will on behalf of the incapable person. This can be done by the Court which tries to place itself in the person's position and leave his/her property, in so far as possible, as s/he would have done.

The problems with this mechanism have been exposed by Gostin. They centre on expense and time. The court is necessarily relatively bureaucratic. Since all sides have to be considered, decisions on major expenditure can take a long time to be made. This may well be to the detriment of the person whose property is being looked after. It has also been an expensive procedure. Indeed it has been unlikely to be financially sensible to involve the Court where the person has less than £5,000 or property to that value. The Court does look after considerable sums of money and concern has been expressed over its investment policies which may have caused people to lose money.

Some of these problems have been overcome. It is now possible to appoint the Public Trustee as the receiver. (See Public Trustee and Administration of Estates Act 1986.) This is an office which is used to dealing with many relatively small sums of money, which is used to taking decisions and has sensible investment practices. The Court of Protection is keen to respond to imaginative means of spending a patient's money for the patient's benefit (see Macfarlane, A., in Carson, D. (ed.) *Making the most of the Court of Protection*, 1987). The service though still has to be paid for out of the person's estate. The Public Trustee will not act as receiver in all cases: relatives will still be appointed where possible. Consequently, it is not yet clear whether the system ensures sufficient flexibility in dealing with the problems of the person incapable of making decisions as to his/her property and affairs.

Sexual relationships and sex education

Personal and social relationships are an important aspect of everyone's life. The freedom to have a sexual relationship is a freedom central to the law valuing people as individuals and as members of society. It is here that the law appears to adopt an inflexible approach which emphasises too strongly the need to protect at least some people with mental handicaps from exploitation and abuse.

The Sexual Offences Acts 1956 and 1967 create major obstacles in the way of some people with mental handicaps having sexual relationships. If a person is accurately described as being a 'defective' or, in the context of homosexuality, 'severely mentally handicapped' (which has the same meaning as 'defective'), the law presumes that s/he will be exploited and abused by a sexual relationship and, therefore, makes such a relationship extremely difficult by the creation of specific criminal offences.

Not all people with mental handicaps can be accurately described as being 'defective', which is defined as:

'A state of arrested or incomplete development of mind which includes severe impairment of intelligence and social functioning.'

The intelligence of most people with mental handicaps is not severely impaired. A rough and ready guide would be an IQ of below 50, but IQ tests may be culturally biased and only measure certain forms of intelligence. Therefore, it would be dangerous to assert that someone's intelligence is severely impaired simply on the result of an IQ test. Further, the social functioning of most people with mental handicaps is not severely impaired either. It is not clear exactly what social functioning is, but it probably requires consideration to be given to a person's ability to look after him/herself and to relate with other people.

It should also be realised that there is not necessarily a clear correlation between the professional/clinical use of the phrase 'severe mental handicap' and the legal terms 'defective/severe mental handicap'. Indeed, the Court of Appeal in *R* v. *Hall* (1987) decided that the concept was one of ordinary English language which was for the court to decide. This means that care must be taken with how people are labelled. If a person is labelled as having a severe mental handicap for one purpose, for example, to receive community support services, that is an indicator that s/he is legally a 'defective' for the purpose of the sexual offences legislation. Since most people with mental handicaps cannot be categorised as 'defective', there is no greater restriction on their sexual relationships than those imposed on anyone else. Consequently, the relationship must be consensual, otherwise the man may have raped the woman.

If, however, a person is a 'defective', s/he is not free to engage in a sexual relationship. It is an offence for 'a man to have unlawful sexual intercourse with a woman who is a defective' and it is an offence for a person to indecently assault a 'defective', who is not allowed, by law, to consent to prevent the act being an assault. (See Sexual Offences Act 1956.)

These offences mean, firstly, that a man cannot have sex with a woman who is a 'defective' even if she is consenting and the relationship is a loving one which is not exploitative or abusive of either party. The law appears to impose a blanket restriction. Some protection is provided for the man: he will not be guilty if he did not know and had no reason to suspect that the woman was a 'defective'. This may well be the case if the man is also severely mentally handicapped, but couples may well be aware of the problems that each has. Consequently, this defence does not ensure that all couples who are handicapped can have a sexual relationship when the woman is severely handicapped.

There will be no offence committed if the couple are married, since the sexual intercourse when the couple are married is not 'unlawful'. Paradoxically, the law does not automatically prevent people who have severe mental handicaps from marrying. In fact, getting married is relatively straightforward. All that is necessary is for the person who is to perform the ceremony to be satisfied that the couple are capable of entering into what is legally a relatively simple contract. This they will be able to display by answering the questions asked of them before and during the ceremony. The law, therefore, imposes a blanket restriction on extra-marital sex for a woman who has a severe mental handicap, but does not automatically prevent her getting married, when it is expected that she will have sex with her husband!

These offences mean, secondly, that people who are 'defectives' may not be able legally to receive the benefit of certain types of sex education. Most people discover their own sexuality and by trial and experiment find out about such things as masturbation and sexual intercourse. This form of learning may be particularly difficult for people with severe mental handicaps. It may be that they have difficulty in making the connection between what they see in books, pictures and videos and themselves. For some people, therefore, 'hands on' teaching may become essential.

'Hands on' teaching will involve an 'assault', because either the person will be touched or believe that s/he is to be touched. Anything to do with sex and, particularly, the genitalia would appear, at face value, to be indecent. Most people, of course, consent to such activity and thus there is no assault. The law, however, states that a man or woman who is a 'defective' is not allowed to consent, for example, to be taught masturbation, even if s/he is clearly willing.

It may be, however, that there is no indecent assault in such circumstances. This would be on the basis of arguing that there was, in fact, no indecency. The House of Lords in *R* v. *Court* (1988) indicated that an assault is indecent if 'right-minded persons would consider the conduct indecent or not'.

Teaching masturbation to people who are incapable of learning it without 'hands on' teaching might be thought not to contravene standards of right-minded persons. It might, therefore, be analogous to a vaginal examination by a doctor or midwife for a genuine medical purpose, which would appear not to be an indecent assault. The situations, however, are not entirely analogous. It might further help to establish that 'hands on' teaching was done with a decent motive. It would be necessary to show that the teacher had no prurient interest. The best way, it is suggested, would be by a case conference involving the client, his/her relatives (if possible) and the relevant professionals in which the progress of the individual is discussed within the context of an individualised programme of personal relationships. It must then be considered whether the right time has come for the teaching of masturbation, whether the client wishes to learn and how the teaching is to be done. If 'hands on' teaching cannot be avoided, it must be decided who is to do it, when and how. An emotional relationship must be not established between teacher and pupil: perhaps a man should not teach a woman. These are difficult decisions, the answers to which must vary from case to case.

Having proposed these means of avoiding legal liability, it must be recognised that there is no guarantee that they would be effective. The law does seem to take the view that all people who are 'defectives' will be exploited or abused by sexual relationships and by understanding their own sexuality. This would appear to be a gross over-generalisation. Although it must be recognised that some people are so abused. Sexual abuse can be very difficult to prove. Even so, prosecuting for the sexual offences is the appropriate means of dealing with the problem unless some use can be made of section 127 of the Mental Health Act 1983. However, these are not the only obstacles. If a couple, one of whom is a 'defective', are having a sexual relationship, any help provided by staff may involve the commission of an offence of 'aiding and abetting' the couple to commit an offence. This will be a particular problem when the couple are also physically handicapped and, therefore, require some assistance with the sex act. It may be a problem even if a room is supplied. In the latter situation, it is also a specific offence for anyone involved in the management of premises 'to induce or knowingly suffer a woman who is a defective to be on the premises for the purpose of having unlawful sexual intercourse . . .'.

If the relationship is long-lasting, this offence creates particular problems. It may be possible to argue that the woman is on the premises for the purpose of living there and happens to have sex. However, this seems to be unlikely to succeed, since people can have more than one purpose in what they do. The law, therefore, seems to impose severe restrictions upon people who have severe mental handicaps. Such restrictions also apply to homosexuality.

There may be some consolation in the fact that, if the relationships are not exploitative or abusive, it is unlikely that they will be reported to the police. If they are, there may be no prosecution. These are only practical points, albeit of considerable importance. The law still imposes what may be perceived as insupportable obstacles if people with mental handicaps are to be valued as individuals and members of society and if appropriate sexual expression is accepted as being an important part of any person's life. At present, there is a stark choice: obey the law and deny a person's sexuality or break the law and run the risk of prosecution.

Treatment

If a person with a mental handicap is to be valued, it is important that his/her treatment decisions be respected. If s/he is incapable of taking such decisions, there must be a proper means of providing necessary and appropriate treatment for his/her benefit.

If s/he is a child under 18 and is incapable of taking treatment decisions, parents may take such decisions on behalf of their children. There is, though, the possibility of the child being made a ward of court, by anyone concerned with the parental decision. (See Cretney, S. M., *Principles of Family Law*, Sweet and Maxwell, London, 1984.) The courts then decide what is in the best interests of the child. A good example is to be found in *Re: B (a Minor) (Wardship: Medical Treatment)* (1981). B was born with Down's Syndrome. Her parents did not want her to have a relatively simple operation which would have relieved an intestinal blockage. The court decided that it was in the child's best interests that the operation should go ahead. Suffering from Down's Syndrome was not a sufficient reason in itself to justify the treatment not being given, which would have led to the child's death. On the other hand, the court indicated that:

'(T)here may be cases . . . of severe proved damage where the future is so uncertain and where the life of the child is so bound to be full of pain and suffering that the court might be driven to a different conclusion . . .'.

It would seem that it would take extremely rare circumstances for the court to be driven to a different conclusion. Should this ever be possible?

In recent years the issue of what can be consented to under wardship, and when, has arisen in relation to a proposal to have a girl sterilised. In *Re: B (a Minor) (Sterilisation)* (1987), the House of Lords has decided that the courts have the right to authorise a sterilisation operation on a ward and that the particular girl in question, Jeanette, should be sterilised. The House recognises that in wardship proceedings a court is concerned to decide what is in the best interests of the child. This is a very broad test and it is not surprising to discover, therefore, that it was accepted that a court can, in appropriate circumstances, authorise a sterilisation operation on a ward. If it is thought that sterilisation can never be appropriate, there will be fundamental disagreement with the decision.

The case is of great significance in deciding when sterilisation may be appropriate. It is affirmed that sterilisation is an operation which involves 'the deprivation of a basic human right, namely the right of a woman to reproduce'. It is, therefore, accepted that sterilisation is a last resort operation. The House rejected a distinction between therapeutic and non-therapeutic reasons for sterilisation. This distinction lay at the basis of the decision of the Supreme Court of Canada in *Re:Eve* (1986) that the Canadian courts could not authorise non-therapeutic sterilisation for social purposes on the basis of existing common law powers, but that if such should be possible, legislation was necessary. It may be that legislation is necessary in this country to determine when sterilisation can be carried out, if at all, and what criteria must be taken into account in order to achieve a proper balance.

The House firmly rejected eugenics and population control as reasons justifying the sterilisation of a girl. It would seem that there is an expectation that there will always have to be court authorisation for such an operation. Consequently an independent and impartial tribunal must always be involved in the decision-making.

Clearly, although the case is very important, it is entirely dependent upon its own particular facts. It should, therefore, be regarded as having limited value in providing general guidance. Jeanette was described as having a moderate degree of mental handicap, but very limited intellectual development. Her ability to understand speech was equivalent to that of a six-year-old, but her expressive ability was that of a five-year-old. She had extremes of mood and could become violent and aggressive. She was not, and would not be, capable of taking informed decisions about contraception and sterilisation. She was on a drug, danazole, to control her irregular periods and to relieve pre-menstrual tension. She suffered from epilepsy which was controlled by 'anti-convulsant drugs'. She suffered from obesity, which meant that the side effects of some drugs made them unusable: she had been prescribed Microgynon 30, an oral contraceptive, to control her violence, but this significantly increased her weight. On the basis that Jeanette showed signs of sexual awareness and sexual drive, the risk of pregnancy came to the notice of her mother and the involved professionals.

The medical evidence indicated that Jeanette had no maternal feelings and, indeed, had an antipathy to children. Although she understood the link between pregnancy and babies, she did not understand the link between sexual intercourse and pregnancy and she could care for herself only at the simplest level, which included management of her own menstruation. It was felt that if she gave birth to a child she would have to have it taken away from her, which would not cause her distress. If she became pregnant, there would have to be a termination, although it would be possible that no-one would realise she was pregnant because of her obesity. If she were to go to term, there could not be a natural birth. There would have to be birth by Caesarian section. She would be likely not to leave the resultant wound alone, because she had played with wounds in the past and displayed a high tolerance of pain.

If pregnancy was to be avoided, the options had to be considered. The medical evidence indicated that mechanical means were ruled out because of her limited intelligence and that the choice of drugs was severely limited, because of her need to receive anti-convulsant drugs. Consequently, the medical evidence indicated that the only options were, first:

'Sterilisation by occluding the fallopian tubes which is a relatively minor operation carrying a small degree of risk, a very high degree of protection and minimal side effects.'

The second option was daily administration of the drug progestogen. But this would have to last for about 30 years, there might be difficulty in ensuring that the daily dosage could be given because of violent tendencies, the possible side-effects over a long term of the drugs was unknown and the effectiveness of the course was entirely speculative. If this course was to be followed, there would have to be a trial period of 12 to 18 months. The House saw the dilemma as a choice between one course which was 'safe, certain, but irreversible' and the other which was 'speculative, possibly damaging and requiring discipline over a long period of time from a person of limited intellectual ability'.

In these circumstances, and on the basis of the evidence presented to them, it is perhaps not surprising that the Lords who are not medical or mental handicap experts came to the decision that they did. The case is not, however, free of question marks. It may be that some of these were actually addressed in evidence before the court, but not stated by the judges in their decision. It was said that Jeanette could not be provided with abstract sex education. What alternatives to abstract means of teaching were considered? If she could be taught to deal with her own menstruation could time have been taken to teach/train her about contraception? Were her apparent advances to members of staff and her touching her genitalia really signs of sexual awareness? If so, what were the prospects of her being sexually promiscuous? If none, or low, would that not be relevant in deciding if an irreversible operation should be performed? How wide-ranging was the consideration of alternative drugs? What means of administration were considered? Could long-term contraceptive drugs have been administered by injection? If she was receiving anti-convulsant drugs, her violence could not have been such as to guarantee that treatment could not be provided. What is wrong with being on a contraceptive pill for 30 years: is that not the means of contraception adopted by most couples?

When considering mechanical means, was it made clear that the coil/IUD would not have been a viable alternative? It is difficult to see how her limited intellectual ability would prevent the use of such a means of contraception.

There is some concern that the decision had to be made prior to 20 May, because Jeanette would then be 18 and there might be problems with sterilising her above that age. Her age would not seem to be a sufficient reason for authorising sterilisation, if it was not justifiable on proper grounds. Whilst the court rejected the idea that her age was of any significance, it would seem that one of the reasons why the alternative of progestogen was thought not to be appropriate was because the trial period would end when she was more than 18 years old. Further, questions might be raised about the decision that Jeanette was and would remain incapable of decision-making. What is capacity in the circumstances? How is it to be established? Since the operation was irreversible, this would rather suggest that an operation should be delayed as long as possible: after 18 if necessary.

Although the case is saying that sterilisation should rarely be carried out, it is perhaps questionable whether judges are capable by their background and the nature of the legal system of establishing the correct criteria on which to base such a decision. It is debatable whether it is fair to ask judges to lay down such criteria. It may also be questionable whether the system ensures that all the facts are made available. It would seem appropriate to have the courts (or some similar independent and impartial tribunal) involved in making decisions about children under 18, when they cannot decide for themselves. The proper criteria could be laid down in legislation or by a body of experts created by legislation, the report of which the courts would be bound to observe. The courts, and parties, would then know what issues had to be considered and rejected before sterilisation could be authorised. This would ensure that all the appropriate issues were considered in achieving a proper balance between the competing demands. The scheme could, of course, extend to all types of treatment.

It is now clear that treatment can be provided to people who are 18 and above and who are incapable of consenting to treatment. Undoubtedly, no-one can take treatment decisions on behalf of a person who has reached 18, even if s/he is incapable. Parents and involved professionals cannot legally provide consent.

In a case called *T* v. *T* (1988), the court had to consider whether it could authorise a termination of pregnancy and the sterilisation of a 19-year-old woman with severe mental handicap. Again, it was simply accepted that the person in question was incapable of consenting on her own behalf. This raises the question of whether there should be someone representing the person with mental handicap, not just in the sense of the official solicitor, but with the specific mandate to act as a sort of Devil's Advocate bound to argue against whatever option is proposed. (I am grateful to Mr S. Lee, London University, for putting the idea in this form.) This would ensure that the strength of the proposal is thoroughly tested.

The question of the legality of the termination was not fully considered. The opinion of the two doctors provided under the Abortion Act 1967 seems to have been accepted with little argument. However, the question of whether she should be sterilised was considered in more detail. Ultimately it was decided that she should be sterilised, perhaps by hysterectomy if the termination was performed by a surgical method since such an operation would also provide simple access to the Fallopian tubes.

Similar factual doubts can be raised about this case as have been debated in the Jeanette case. Of more importance is the legal principle laid down which entitled the judge to say that these forms of medical treatment could be performed without the doctors incurring legal liability. The solution that the judge put forward was that the treatment would be lawful if it was in the best interests of the patient's health and was demanded by good medical practice, in the sense that there weren't differing views about the proposed treatment.

Whilst this does provide a solution, it is not entirely satisfactory. It seems to leave the decision in the hands of the treatment provider, since there appears to be no expectation of referral to a court in all instances, except, perhaps in the most intrusive forms of treatment. If the decision is to be taken solely by the treatment provider, it is to be questioned whether the views of the person with a mental handicap are adequately catered for. Much depends upon the integrity and open-mindedness of the treatment provider. It does not allow for those who hold idiosyncratic views and seems to impose an enormous burden on treatment providers, one that they are unlikely to be keen to bear.

Consequently, treatment can be provided for incapable people of all ages. The law is, though, unclear and unsatisfactory if the person is an adult. Too much of a burden is placed on care staff and particularly the doctors involved. If people with mental handicaps are to be valued properly, there should be a mechanism for allowing a court to appoint a person to take treatment decisions on behalf of adults, but s/he should be responsible to a court to examine the appropriateness of those decisions. This would appear to be demanded by the United Nations Declaration on the Rights of Mentally Retarded Persons in article 5:

> 'The mentally retarded person has a right to a qualified guardian when this is required to protect his personal well-being and interests.'

It is possible that the House of Lords may encourage this possibility, because Lord Oliver accepted that a court has the power to take treatment decisions on the basis of the historical parens patriae power of the courts ('Father of the state/people'). This is somewhat surprising since it has been assumed that no such power exists now, even if it did in the past. Further, whether the power exists or not was not fully or properly considered. Consequently, no-one would know how to exercise such a power; there is no known procedure for exercising it. Whilst it is an exciting suggestion which could resolve the problem, it would appear to be preferable to adopt a legislative scheme to ensure that the UN demand is properly fulfilled for both adults and children.

Education

Education is crucial to anyone's development. The valuing process would aim to ensure that each person fulfils his/her potential if at all possible. His/her individual needs must be recognised and responded to. The Education Act 1981 appears to fulfil this requirement.

The Act requires that the special educational needs of all children with learning difficulties be assessed by the local education authority. If the assessment indicates that some special provision is necessary, it is for the LEA in its discretion to decide whether such provision can be made in ordinary schools or whether it is necessary to go further and be more specific by making a statement of the special educational provision that should be made for the child. The formal process involves not only the LEA and its officers, but also teachers, experts (psychological, medical, etc.) and the child's parents.

This appears to be a flexible response to the needs of the individual child. However, the LEA is only required and empowered to make *educational* provision. The statement may include a reference to essential *non-educational* provision. This might suggest the provision of speech therapy. Speech therapy is not the responsibility of LEAs, but of district health authorities. Can the LEA be required to supply speech therapy or at least be required to pay for it?

These questions were posed in *R. v. Oxfordshire County Council, ex parte AGW* (1986). The court decided that, particularly in the light of the history of speech therapy, it was not irrational or unreasonable for the LEA to describe speech therapy as non-educational provision and therefore it did not have a duty to supply this service. The court then considered that the LEA did not have the power to pay for speech therapy. Even though it may be clear that speech therapy is essential to a child's development, a LEA cannot provide it or pay for it and there is no duty on the district health authority to provide speech therapy. In fact, in this case the health authority did agree to provide speech therapy. So, a child may not be provided with an essential service unless the health authority decides to spend money on an extensive speech therapy service, which may be at the expense of other health care provision. Therefore, a child's potential will not necessarily be maximised. Too much depends upon the commitment of the various authorities and the vagaries of finance and resources.

Provision of welfare services

Many services, particularly welfare services, essential to the proper lifestyle of a person with a mental handicap are provided at the discretion of some authorities. There is considerable dependence upon the individual being able to argue that s/he should be provided with a particular service. This means that s/he must be able to present an argument to the local social services authority. Many people with mental handicaps will find this difficult if not impossible.

Progress will be made when the Disabled Persons (Services, Consultation and Representation) Act 1986 comes into force. It will allow people to be appointed to represent the views of handicapped and other disabled people who cannot represent themselves at meetings which are to decide upon the provision of welfare services. It is not clear, however, when this Act will be brought into force and it is limited in its scope. It should, though, provide some impetus to the call for advocacy services so that the voice of people with mental handicaps can be heard where it matters.

Conclusion

This brief review of some aspects of the law as it affects people with mental handicaps would appear to indicate that the law has not achieved the correct balance referred to at the outset. It would not appear consistently to ensure that such people are valued as individuals and as members of society. Indeed, much the same exercise with the same result could be undertaken in other areas of the law, particularly in relation to the provision of accommodation in both the public and private sectors and the criminal justice system.

Much more specific thought needs to be given to the needs of people with mental handicaps. It is not appropriate to discuss these needs with the needs of other groups. Perhaps the time has come for legislation. This may happen as a result of the public debate over the Jeanette and *T* v. *T* cases. Any legislation should not be limited to treatment decisions, where a full-blown guardianship system would certainly be advantageous, but consideration should be given to extensive guardianship to allow proper decisions to be taken in all spheres, but only where the individual is incapable of that type of decision.

Provided any system of guardianship was sufficiently flexible, it might be possible to assert that the balance between independence and protection was at last being achieved and the demands of the United Nations Declaration on the Rights of Mentally Retarded Persons was being fulfilled.

Further reading

1. Gostin, L. O., *The Court of Protection* (Mind, London, 1983).
2. Whitehorn, N., *Court of Protection Handbook* (Longman Professionals, 7th edition, 1985).
3. Carson, D., (ed.) *Making the Most of the Court of Protection* (King's Fund Centre, London, 1987).

4. Article 8 of the *European Convention on Human Rights* and Gunn, M. J., 'Human Rights and Mental Handicap', *Mental Handicap*, vol. 14 (1986).
5. Sexual Offences Act 1956 as amended by Mental Health (amendment) Act 1982.
6. For some tests on social functioning, see Gilbert, P., *Mental Handicap: A Practical Guide for Social Workers* (Business Press International, Sutton, Surrey, 1985).
7. Gunn, M. J., with Rosser, J., *Sex and the Law: A Brief Guide for Staff Working in the Mental Handicap Field* (Family Planning Association, London, 1987).
8. 31 Dominion Law Reports, 4th series, 1986.
9. *Marshall* v. *Curry* (1933) 3 Dominion Law Reports 260; *Murray* v. *McMurchy* (1949) 2 Dominion Law Reports 442; and Hoggett, B. M., *Mental Health Law* (Sweet and Maxwell, 2nd edition, 1984).
10. Gunn, M. J., *Treatment and Mental Handicap* (1987); 16 *Anglo-American Law Review* 242 and Gunn, M. J. Note on *T* v. *T* (1988) *Journal of Social Welfare Law* (forthcoming).
11. Education Act 1981, for meaning of learning difficulty and special educational needs see Section 1.
12. See *R* v. *Secretary of State for Education and Science, ex parte Lashford, The Independent*, 13 May 1987.
13. National Assistance Act 1948, National Health Service Act 1977 and Chronically Sick and Disabled Persons Act 1970.
14. Herr, S. S., *Rights and Advocacy for Retarded People* (Lexington Books, 1983).

PART TWO

A life in the community

CHAPTER 4

Educational policy, legislation and implementation: the impact of the 1981 Education Act

Peter Farrell
Co-tutor MSC Educational Training Course, University of Manchester

One central objective of the 1981 Education Act was the introduction of a system of identification, assessment and review of all children with special educational needs which was fully accountable to parents, which involved a prescribed group of professionals and which was placed within a legal framework. Although the Act covers many aspects of special education, it is the formal assessment procedures, sometimes referred to as the 'statementing' or Section Five Assessment Procedures, which have had the greatest impact on LEA practice in England and Wales.

As the Act has been in force since April 1983 and its detailed provisions are well known, these will not be repeated here. However, in relation to the formal assessment procedures, the following key features are worth re-emphasising. First, as stated above, the Act provides a legal framework for the formal assessment of children who may have special educational needs who will require 'provision additional to, or otherwise different from, the facilities and resources generally available in ordinary schools in the area under normal arrangements' (DES, 1983b para. 13). These children are thought to correspond to those who were in special schools when the Act was drafted. Second, it ensures that assessment is multi-disciplinary, involving at the very least a teacher, an educational psychologist and a school doctor. (For children with severe learning difficulties, other professionals including paediatricians, social workers, speech therapists and physiotherapists will often be involved.) Third, the procedures actively seek the involvement of parents, by requiring formal agreement to an assessment going ahead and making it possible for parents to request an LEA to conduct an assessment. Parents can also present their own views on the child, which should be given equal weighting to the professional's views, and they can collect 'evidence' from professionals consulted independently. Furthermore, parents see the draft and final statements of the child's special educational needs which the LEA compiles and which include all the reports from the different professionals involved and they have a right to appeal against the provision outlined for their child in the statement. Fourth, the Act lays down procedures for the annual review of statements and for the formal re-assessments which occur when the child reaches the age of 13½, the so-called 'Thirteen Plus Review'.

Many excellent summaries of the Act have been produced which go into far greater detail than there is space for here, for example, the handbook produced by the Advisory Council for Education, ACE (1983). In addition most LEAs in England and Wales have written summaries for professionals and parents. These often include flow diagrams which are designed to simplify the formal assessment procedures of the Act. However, the Act itself, DES (1981a); the Regulations, DES (1983a); and the accompanying circulars – Circular 8/81, DES (1981b), and Circular 1/83, DES (1983b) – provide the most comprehensive coverage of the Act and its provisions.

To date several authors have commented about the effects of the 1981 Education Act, see for example Russell (undated), Bookbinder (1983a, b), Self (1983) Kerfoot and Gray (1984), Peter (1984), Wedell *et al.* (1982). In addition, several LEAs have conducted their own surveys on the ways it has been implemented, for example, Chandler (1986) and the Derbyshire Survey (1984), while Vaughan (1986) surveyed all LEAs in England and Wales and the National Council for Special Education have commissioned their own enquiry. Finally, the results of a major DES project are now available: Wedell *et al.* (1976). This three-year project looked in detail at the procedures for assessing and making provision for children with special educational needs and was conducted by a team from the University of London Institute of Education (ULIE). Recently the House of Commons Select Committee into the implementation of the 1981 Act, which has been collecting evidence from individuals, professional associations, LEAs, institutes of higher education and voluntary agencies, published its findings (House of Commons, 1987).

In the sections which follow, the implications of formal assessment procedures on services for children with special educational needs will be considered, with an emphasis on children with severe learning difficulties. The sections cover the implications for parents, professionals and administrators. The research conducted by ULIE and the findings of the House of Commons enquiry will be referred to on a number of occasions.

Implications for parents

One positive effect of the 1981 Act has been the closer involvement of parents in the assessment of their children and this development can be seen as part of a wider movement to involve parents in all aspects of their children's education. In the field of mental handicap, these developments have been going on for some time (see, for example, Cunningham and Jeffree, 1971; Cameron, 1979; Mittler and McConachie, 1983). However, in regard to the detailed ways in which parents are involved in formal assessments, the following important issues still need to be resolved.

How should parents make their views known to the LEA?

The 1981 Act and Circular 1/83 do not provide any guidelines or suggestions as to how parents should represent their views on their child to the LEA. The absence of guidelines was a serious omission, as for many parents it is the first time that they will have been asked to write a description of their child's difficulties. This can be a daunting task for many parents, who, while wishing to contribute to their child's assessment, may nevertheless have difficulty in putting their thoughts on paper, particularly at the potentially sensitive time when their child is to undergo a complex assessment procedure involving a range of different professionals.

Fortunately, since the Act came into force, several initiatives have taken place where guidelines to help parents present their views have been developed. See Wolfendale (1985) for a well-known example. Currently it appears that few LEAs are using such guidelines on a regular basis. In fact the ULIE research found that only 28% of LEAs said that all or most of their parents contributed advice to the statement either using guidelines or by writing their own comments independently. However, in one small study (Chandler, 1986), 36 parents of children with a range of special educational needs on whom statements had recently been completed where shown a copy of the Wolfendale guidelines, and 83% of this sample reported that they would have found them very useful in helping them to make their views known about their child. It is to be hoped that LEAs will encourage parents to use such guidelines more often in the future.

Evidence supplied by parents

In addition to the parents' own views on their child, they are invited to provide written evidence from professionals whom they may have consulted independently. From what is known about the way the Act has been implemented, it appears that very few, if any, parents are using their right to gain such evidence. The ULIE research and the very full evidence to the House of Commons enquiry from the Voluntary Council for Handicapped Children (1987) provide no figures as to the number of parents who have supplied independent evidence on behalf of their child. One problem is that there is precious little machinery available in Local

Authorities for parents to collect 'independent' evidence, unless they can afford to pay for a private assessment, and even then the availability of private agencies varies considerably throughout the country. In any case, such agencies may be unable to complete a thorough assessment as they do not always have access to the settings in which the child functions: for example, the nursery and/or assessment unit. Consequently the only appropriate person to carry out an independent assessment may be an employee of the LEA where the parents live, but because of his or her status as an employee, the parents may justifiably believe that this assessment cannot be truly independent.

In regard to independent psychological advice, the British Psychological Society and the Association of Educational Psychologists have suggested that if parents do not wish to use another psychologist from the LEA where they live they should be allowed to approach an educational psychologist from a neighbouring authority. However, very few requests of this kind have been made. The Advisory Council for Education (ACE) has also set up an independent panel of professional experts on whom they can call when parents request an independent assessment but it is possible that not all LEA personnel are aware that such a panel exists.

Unfortunately therefore, the position regarding parents being able to provide independent evidence is still uncertain and it is hoped that the problems outlined above can be quickly overcome so that this well-intentioned provision of the 1981 Act can be made *freely* available to parents who wish to use it.

The role of the 'named person'

The 1981 Education Act accepted, in part, the Warnock Committee's recommendation that parents should be given the name of a person whom they could consult throughout the assessment process. Unfortunately the Act does not lay down who the named person(s) should be at any of the stages when his or her name is given to the parents (i.e., when notification is served and when the draft and final statements are delivered). Nor does Circular 1/83 specify what the person's role should be, other than one of providing more information about any part of the statementing procedures. Russell (undated) has written in some detail about the potential role of the named person and suggests that it should be a person who may act in the capacity of a parent advocate while at the same time working to ensure that the LEA is using its resources effectively. She also suggests that these people should be trained for such a role and after considering the advantages and disadvantages of different professionals within an LEA fulfilling this function, she suggests that volunteers could be trained to perform this task in the same way that training is provided for lay justices.

Clearly Russell sees the role of the named person to go far beyond the narrow 'information-providing' brief which is implied in Circular 1/83. These views are reinforced by the evidence to the House of Commons enquiry by the Voluntary Council for Handicapped Children (1987) which stresses the potential role of voluntary agencies in providing the named person as a 'parent befriender'. However, the ULIE research found that only 17% of LEAs held regular meetings with voluntary agencies about the 1981 Act and they did not on the whole consider these agencies as suppliers of named people. Indeed, the ULIE research showed that LEAs had accepted the guidelines in Circular 1/83 and use educational administrators as named people seeing their role not as child advocates or befrienders but as clarifiers of the procedures. Few parents appear to consult their LEA officer for this purpose, preferring to discuss these issues with the professionals who are conducting the assessment.

Appeals

Parents can formally appeal at two distinct stages and for different reasons. Firstly, they can appeal direct to the Secretary of State if an LEA decides, against the parents' wishes, not to proceed with an assessment. The ULIE figures show that the DES had ruled in favour of the parents in only 10% of appeals of this kind.

Secondly, parents can appeal to the LEA against the provision specified in the statement and if they are dissatisfied with the outcome they can appeal direct to the Secretary of State. The ULIE research showed that 73% of appeals to the LEA were unsuccessful and in the 27% of successful cases, where the Local Appeals Committee had requested that an LEA reconsider the provision, over one-third of the LEAs did not comply. Of the few parents who took the matter further by appealing to the Secretary of State, only 27% were successful in persuading the DES to ask the LEA to amend the statement.

On the whole, this evidence suggests that parents who appeal are usually unsuccessful. The following reasons for this have been suggested. First, the LEA appeals panels are overwhelmingly made up of LEA officers, a point made by the Law Society Group for the Welfare of People with a Mental Handicap (1985). Second, it seems unfair that parents can only appeal against the provision in a statement and not against its overall conclusions or against the findings of the individual advice givers. This restricts their freedom to discuss wider issues. Third, the appeals procedures are extremely cumbersome and time-consuming and this in itself may result in issues which were crucial at the time the statement was delivered seeming less important when the appeal is heard.

Whatever happened to partnership?

Apart from the specific issues of parents' representations and evidence, their use of the named person and the appeals procedure, which are discussed above, the whole ethos of the 1981 Education Act is one of promoting effective partnerships between parents and professionals. Has this occurred? Unfortunately the evidence suggests that parents are dissatisfied with many features of the statutory procedures and that we still have some way to go before achieving the goal of effective partnership. The House of Commons enquiry, the ULIE research and Rogers (1986) all suggest that parents are concerned about the following features of the Act: first, the documentation is complex and not always easy to understand particularly for families from ethnic minorities whose understanding of English may be limited; second, the parents' views and evidence are not given equal weighting to the professionals' advice; and third, the eventual outcome of the assessment may be decided at the start and little opportunity is given to parents to explore alternative outcomes, particularly those involving some form of integration.

Evans (1987) in her summary of the ULIE Research Project concludes by stating: 'It was difficult for both sides to achieve the "partnership" envisaged by the Act. Parents were inhibited by their lack of knowledge and support: officers and professionals by their lack of time and resources' (p.16). Finally in the evidence to the House of Commons enquiry, MENCAP (1987) make the point that parents are the only group whose views on the child have to be submitted within a time limit (29 days). Such constraints on one group of advice givers hardly reflects the spirit of partnership which is supposedly embodied by the Act.

Implications for professional practice

This section considers three areas of professional practice which are causing concern: the co-ordination of services, the variations in provision which may be offered and the quality of the professionals' advice.

The co-ordination of services

One central feature of the statementing procedure is the emphasis on multi-disciplinary assessment. For children with severe learning difficulties, who are almost always identified in the first few years of life, the responsibility for instigating the assessment procedures lies with the District Health Authorities who, under Section 10 of the Act, are required to refer children who may have special educational needs to the LEA so that Section Five Assessment Procedures can be initiated. However, the ULIE research showed that there were wide variations in the way the District Health Authorities and LEAs co-ordinated their activities and that in many cases children with severe learning difficulties were not being referred soon enough. Indeed, it was rare for LEAs and Health Authorities to have an agreed and co-ordinated plan with which to identify and assess pre-school children with special educational needs.

Some areas of the country have well-established district handicap teams, often based at Child Development Centres in hospitals, where all the relevant professionals can meet and conduct a truly multi-disciplinary assessment. For children with severe learning difficulties this co-ordination of services is essential, since they frequently need the expertise of a range of professionals, including speech therapists, physiotherapists and social workers. All these services can usually be provided at a Child Development Centre. This facilitates communication between all parties, including the parents, and reduces the burden which many parents face of having to trail their children to different hospitals and clinics in order to see a number of professionals, whose services may be poorly co-ordinated.

In addition to Child Development Centres, LEAs could extend the Portage type home-visiting schemes. A few LEAs employ pre-school home visitors and others have successfully bid for money to support a Portage home-visiting project. In view of the success of these schemes it would be advantageous for all LEAs to appoint specially trained home visitors who can be a vital resource to families in helping them through the difficult period of coming to terms with having a child with severe learning difficulties, and in giving them skills to work with their child. They could also play a crucial role in liaising with all the professionals in the Child Development Centres who are involved in the formal assessment process.

It is clearly vital for LEAs and Health Authorities to co-ordinate their activities so that children with special educational needs are referred at the appropriate time to the relevant agencies, possibly through a well-resourced Child Development Centre or a pre-school home visitor.

The range of provision

Although the 1981 Education Act did not explicitly instruct LEAs to increase the range of integrated provision, the implication in Circular 1/83 is that statemented children should attend ordinary schools wherever possible. However, it appears that practice on integration varies considerably between LEAs. An increasing number are placing young children with Down's Syndrome in ordinary school with varying degrees of support. Others have a range of units attached to mainstream schools enabling locational, social and some functional integration to take place: see Farrell and Sugden (1985); Mittler and Farrell (in press). Currently no LEA has developed a co-ordinated policy for the long-term integration of children with severe learning difficulties and consequently the range of provision offered to parents varies considerably depending on where they live. However, even in LEAs which can provide integrated facilities for young children with severe learning difficulties, the vast majority end up in special schools by the time they reach junior school age.

The ULIE research suggests that parents' wishes for integrated provision were not always taken into account by professionals who seemed to be steering the children towards special schools, possibly because this was consistent with LEA provision. This was a particular danger in the LEAs who used 'assessment placements' by arranging for a child to attend a special school or unit on an interim basis pending completion of an assessment. In these cases some parents felt the decision about the long-term future education of their child had been decided *before* a full assessment had been carried out and that once a school had 'got its claws' on a child it was reluctant to let go. The Voluntary Council for Handicapped Children (1987) has suggested that one way round this problem would be to formally re-assess pre-school children who have been statemented when they reach school age.

However, these problems would not be so acute if, as suggested above, LEAs appointed home visitors who could ensure that services were well-co-ordinated. The need for assessment placements would then be reduced, although children might attend local nurseries and play groups with support from, or co-ordinated by, the home-visiting teacher.

The divided loyalties of professionals

Clearly one of the difficulties faced by LEA personnel when conducting their assessments is that their detailed knowledge of LEA provision may influence how they relate to parents and how they write their advice. Many professionals may wish to take on the role of parent advocate and make recommendations for facilities and resources to meet a child's needs in the full knowledge that the LEA doesn't have the provision to meet these needs. However, it may be counter-productive to do this as parents' hopes may be raised and then dashed and the whole assessment process may become very long and drawn out. Furthermore some professionals may not wish to risk the possibility of upsetting their administrators by making recommendations which the LEA cannot meet and at the same time increasing the hostility of the parents to the LEA. Indeed there is some evidence from the ULIE research that parents felt that the professionals were meeting the needs of the LEA and not those of the children by making recommendations to suit existing provision.

The quality of the professionals' advice

Quite apart from the issue of whether the professionals' advice matches the LEA provision, some concern has been expressed in the ULIE data about the quality of advice generally. This has tended to be very general, non-specific and not helpful to the parents or to the child's future teachers in terms of helping them to implement an individual educational programme.

The role of professionals in writing advice is not an easy one. Teachers and psychologists in particular would like to help those who will eventually work with the child to plan and carry out an effective educational programme. However one doubts whether including such detail in the advice would be very helpful, partly because statements take a long time to complete and hence written programmes would be out of date when they are delivered, and partly because Circular 1/83 suggests that it should be the teacher who eventually works with the child who should plan a detailed programme of work. Consequently advice tends to be general and only helpful to the LEA in providing them with evidence on which to make a decision about a child's placement.

Clearly teachers and psychologists need to use alternative ways to provide suggestions about educational programmes to the parents and staff who work with a child with special educational needs. Such advice is better given in consultation with those who work with the child including, if possible, the child him/herself. This enables programmes to be tried out, modified and adapted.

Implications for LEA administrators

One of the central findings of the House of Commons enquiry was that LEAs have had considerable problems coping with the administrative procedures associated with the implementing of the statementing process. The length of time taken for statements to be completed varies considerably. In the West Midlands' LEAs the average time between notification and the statement varies from an average of five months in one LEA to 13 months in another. In one LEA in the North West the administrators have predicted that for the academic year 1987/88 the average length of time between serving notice of intention to assess a child and the completion of the statement will be 33 months!

The ULIE research showed that LEAs find the procedures cumbersome and over-bureaucratic and that they 'cut across good practice'. The House of Commons enquiry has recommended that the DES investigate ways of making the procedures more streamlined by, for example, setting time limits for the receipt of professionals' reports and a time limit of about six months for the completion of statements. Whether this can be achieved successfully without LEAs employing more administrators and professionals is open to doubt. There is certainly a need to identify those LEAs who seem to be 'on top' of the procedures and disseminate this good practice to other areas of the country.

Conclusion

This chapter has highlighted some of the problems and issues which have arisen following the implementation of the 1981 Education Act. Inevitably many of these apply to all children with special educational needs but where appropriate, issues concerned with the assessment of children with severe learning difficulties have been considered. Although the House of Commons enquiry stresses everyone's belief that the Act has brought many benefits to families and children with special educational needs, particularly in terms of ensuring the comprehensive multi-disciplinary assessment of children and the involvement of parents, criticisms have been made concerning the way it has been implemented. First, many parents find the whole statementing procedure very complex and difficult to understand. Second, the administrative procedures seem over-bureaucratic and time-consuming. Third, the various professional services are poorly co-ordinated. Fourth, there is a wide variety in the range of provision which different LEAs offer with some LEAs placing pre-school children with severe learning difficulties in ordinary schools with support from specially-trained staff, while other LEAs place all children with special educational needs in special schools. Finally, there appears to be a conflict of interests among many professionals who are torn between being active parent advocates making recommendations for facilities and resources which the LEA cannot provide, or trying to persuade the parents to accept the limited provision which an LEA can offer and which may only partially meet the needs of the child.

In 1985 the government rejected proposals to form a National Advisory Committee for Special Education, which could advise the Government on all issues related to children with special educational needs. However, the House of Commons enquiry has bowed to increased pressure and has re-affirmed the need for the formation of a monitoring group which would concentrate on features of the Act which are causing problems and encourage LEAs to find ways of overcoming them. Whether such a group would fulfil all the functions envisaged in the original proposal for a National Advisory Committee is hard to tell, but given the problems which have been highlighted by this chapter, the need for a centrally-organised body to take substantial steps to improve services to children with special educational needs has never been greater.

Further reading

1. ACE, *Education Act 1981* (Advisory Centre for Education, London, 1983).
2. Bookbinder, 'A New Deal or Dashed Hopes?', *Special Education: Forward Trends,* vol. 10, 1983 No. 1, pp. 6–7.
3. Cameron, R. J., (ed.) *Working Together: Portage in the UK* (NFER-Nelson, 1982).
4. Chandler, L., *The Implementation of the 1981 Education Act: Parents' Perceptions of the Statementing Procedure* (M.Sc. Thesis, Department of Education, University of Manchester, 1986).
5. Cunningham, C., Jeffree, P., *Working with Parents: Developing a Course for Young Mentally Handicapped Children* (London, National Society for the Mentally Handicapped Child, 1971).
6. DES (1981a) *Education Bill* (HMSO).
7. DES (1981b) *Education Act 1981* (Circular 8/81).
8. DES (1983a) *The Education (Special Needs) Regulations 1983.*
9. DES (1983b) *Assessments and Statements of Special Educational Needs* (Circular 1/83).
10. Derbyshire County Council (1985), *Meeting Special Educational Needs in Derbyshire.*
11. Evans, J., *Decision-Making for Special Needs* (University of London Institute of Education, 1987).
12. Farrell, P., Sugden, M., 'Integrating Children with Severe Learning Difficulties. Fantasy or Reality?', *Educational and Child Psychology*, vol. 2, 1985, 3.69–80.
13. Goucher, B., Evans, J., Welton, J., and Wedell, K., *Policy and provisions for special educational needs* (Cassell, 1987).
14. House of Commons, *Special Educational Needs: Implementation of The Education Act 1981,* vol. I & II, 1987, HMSO.
15. Kerfoot, S., Gray, P., 'Humanizing the 1981 Education Act' *Newsletter of the Division of Educational and Child Psychology, British Psychological Society*, vol. 16, 1984, 20–2.
16. Law Society Group for the Welfare of People with a Mental Handicap (1985) *Discussion Paper on the 1981 Education Act.*
17. MENCAP, 'Evidence to the House of Commons Enquiry'. *House of Commons Special Educational Needs. The Implementation of the 1981 Education Act,* vol. II, 1987, HMSO.
18. Mittler, P., McConachie, I., (eds.) *Parents, Professionals and Mentally Handicapped People: Approaches to Partnership* (Croom Helm, 1983).
19. Mittler, P., Farrell, P., (in press) 'Can Children with Severe Learning Difficulties Be Educated in Ordinary Schools?', to appear in the *European Journal of Special Education.*

20. Peter, M., 'A Hard Act to Follow', *Times Educational Supplement*, 30 March 1984.
21. Rogers, R., *Caught in the Act* (Centre for Studies on Integration in Education (CSIE), 1986).
22. Russell, 'The Education Act 1981: The Role of the Named Person', *Early Child Development and Care,* vol. 19, 1985, pp.251–74.
23. Selfe, L., 'Integration and the 1981 Education Act – A Conflict of Interests', *Education Psychology in Practice*, vol. 1, 1985, 1, pp. 14–19.
24. Vaughan, M., *Caught in the Act – What LEAs Tell Parents Under the 1981 Education Act* (Centre for Studies on Integration in Education, 1986).
25. Wolfendale, S., 'Parental Profiling and the Parental Contribution to Section 5 (Education Act 1981). Assessment and Statementing Procedures', *Newsletter of the Association for Child Psychology and Child Psychiatry*, vol. 7, 1985, 2, pp.16–19.
26. Voluntary Council for Handicapped Children, 'Evidence to the House of Commons Enquiry', *House of Commons Special Educational Needs, The Implementation of the 1981 Education Act*, vol. I, 1987, HMSO.
27. Wedell, K., Welton, J., Vorhaus, G., 'Challenges of the 1981 Act', *Special Education: Forward Trends.* vol. 2, 1982 p.608.
28. Wedell, K., Goucher, B., Welton, J., Evans, J., *The 1981 Education Act: Policy and Provision for Special Educational Needs* (Unpublished Report to the Department of Education and Science, University of London, Institute of Education, 1986).

CHAPTER 5

Pre-school and school support

J. E. Buggy
*Specialist Senior Social Worker, Manchester Social Services
Department*

In recent times we have seen a shift from traditional hostel provision,
for handicapped people, to more local and more family-type
settings. Examples of these are: staffed group homes, flats, minimum support homes, long-term fostering and respite fostering,
domiciliary carers and a variety of *ad hoc* schemes throughout the
country.

The latest Government initiative has encouraged this development, particularly care away from the large, outmoded long-stay
mental handicap hospitals and with the emphasis on handicap as an
educational or developmental, rather than a medical, problem there
have been many positive initiatives in this area. In one such area the
city of Manchester has made some useful strides.

In this particular chapter the contents reflect the practices currently carried out by Manchester Social Services Department (and
incorporate future trends in service provision nationally), namely
respite fostering, carers, long-term fostering, short-term care and
playschemes for profoundly retarded and multiply handicapped
people.

The city of Manchester is divided into six social work areas each
with a specialist social work team, specialising in work with
mentally handicapped people. These teams are backed up by a
specialist social work team which is centrally based, covering the
whole city, and basically provides resources in the form of short-
term care, long-stay care, residential provision, respite fostering,
some long-stay fostering and playschemes. The team comprises
three social workers, one of them a senior worker. The senior
social worker is a team leader and works mainly with the residential
units whereas the two Level III social workers primarily work on
the respite fostering programme. The team's primary focus is on
children with severe learning difficulties, who are of school age,
but as chronology means so little in this particular area, it is merely
used as a guideline.

The role of the family support unit

The family support unit is usually a purpose-built home/hostel or an ordinary house in the community with qualified residential social work staff, i.e., houseparents. Respite fostering is another form of family support and some local authorities have carers available to actually go into a family's home to allow the parents/family some time off. This latter form of relief is gaining support as one of its advantages is that the handicapped person does not have to leave home.

A definition

In the context of this chapter, short-term care refers to the arrangements whereby a handicapped child is looked after in a place other than his or her home for a period of time which includes at least one night but does not exceed two or three months.

Philosophy

The philosophy of the family support unit is to provide care for the children and give relief to the parents and family of those who are severely mentally handicapped. The policy is to treat the child first and the handicap second, to make the transition from home to the support unit as smoothly as possible and to make the new living environment of the child as close to the home environment as is feasible. This can only be done by staff getting to know the child well so that a gradual introduction can be made.

Procedures for Admission

These procedures apply to all children who attend special schools, now known as schools for children with severe learning difficulties, and within an approximate age range of between two and 19 years. Referrals are sent to the Central Specialist Social Work Section which is the home-finding team for handicapped children. Once the referral is received the child will then be visited either at home or at school, though more usually this initial visit is to the school. An assessment of the child is made in the school with the teacher observing the child and making notes. Following this a written report is compiled and a copy given to the social worker, the family and to the school. A set of papers including the assessment is then presented to the residential units/respite-giver and a visit is made to the child in the specialist school by a member of the special unit staff, accompanied by the respite care organiser. The visit is usually in the early stages of the procedure.

The family are then asked to visit the residential unit, if they are able. The respite care organiser and residential unit staff then visit the family in the home and it is also generally preferable if the family and the child can visit the residential unit prior to any introduction of the child. Introductions can then take the form of a few hours in the unit, perhaps half a day, leading up to a stay overnight and eventually a weekend stay. The residential unit staff compile a written report following the first-night stay of the child and usually comment on how the child has settled and the suitability of the unit for the child and vice versa. When the child is settled and all those concerned agree to the placement, the family or field social worker arrange subsequent periods of care, whichever is the more appropriate, though it is better if one particular person is given the task to organise the care which will eliminate confusion and duplication and also keep the amount of bureaucracy to a minimum.

The support unit staff continue to pay occasional visits to the child at home and in school. This is to get to know the child better and learn how best to handle them when in care. It is also done to aid continuity, especially if behaviour modification training programmes are required to help maintain the child at a particular functioning level. It also helps to break down barriers between the residential units and family. These inevitably occur from time to time, particularly as the family may feel inadequate about being unable to continue to care for the child and may find it a brief embarrassment each time they visit the residential unit.

There are factors regarding admission which sometimes arise which one cannot control: for example family illness, lack of extended family support, clients' desire to continue caring for the child in family circumstances, even though the pressure of doing so may be taking its toll.

There is also another factor which needs observation and scrutiny. The support unit can be very easily seen as a 'cure' for all the family's problems, leading to a request for an increase in short-term care. It takes a very close and detailed approach to work with the family by the social worker, to be able to see this and particularly do something about it. Indiscriminate and unthinking use of short-term care can obscure deep-seated emotional problems within the family and may require the type of intervention described above. In other words, too many professionals can often overlook the real problem in a family by doling out short-term care on an *ad hoc* basis. Therefore the aims/goals in working with the family must involve close co-operation and a clear, well worked out, easily achieved plan for all the family. The need for a constant assessment of the family's needs is uppermost in achieving the goals. In other words there are levels or thresholds of coping: a particular family with a relatively able handicapped child may need more care/respite than another family with a profoundly retarded and multiply handicapped child. In some cases the fact that respite can be given on a short notice basis can be sufficient, knowing that they will get a break when they want it.

Respite fostering

Another increasingly popular form of family support is the respite foster parent. The respite care scheme which began in 1979 offers relief to parents of mentally handicapped children on an occasional or regular basis, depending on need. Procedures for the use of foster parents are basically the same as those used when placing a child in the family support unit.

Specially recruited foster parents are available to receive handicapped young children into their own home for limited periods, so giving parents some free time, whilst simultaneously providing the children with an enjoyable and useful experience of living temporarily somewhere other than home. Experience has suggested that a successful single period of respite care frequently develops into a more regular arrangement between natural parents and foster parents, so providing the handicapped youngsters with a home away from home, whilst avoiding drawing on the resources of residential or hospital care.

The children

The criteria for placing a child on this is similar to the one used for placing the child in a residential unit for short-term care, for by and large the children on this scheme tend to be younger, though the range of handicap is broad. Where there is more than one mentally handicapped child in the family, brothers and sisters can be accommodated together. Most of the children on the scheme live permanently at home, but there are also some who are at residential schools for much of the year, for whom some respite care can be offered during school holidays, and some children are fostered on a long-term basis.

The foster parents

The foster parents are all formally approved by the Department of Social Services and will have shown particular interest in helping mentally handicapped children. Many have brought up families already and some have a working experience with mentally handicapped children. Maturity, warmth and resilience are particularly desired qualities in this area of work and age is a secondary consideration.

Advantages of respite care

The advantages of respite care are many. The primary one is that the child is still able to live at home with the family. In the past children were admitted to long-term residential care, whether in hospital or long-stay residential units, if an authority had a facility. This meant that only a limited number of people were able to receive some form of support. Nowadays we find a more purposeful plan being drawn up for the handicapped child which includes the role of the family support unit. The permutations of this unit are many. The child can be left there for a couple of hours while the family does some shopping, the family can call to see the staff and talk about ways of coping with the child, perhaps in relation to toilet training etc. This then makes the family support unit a more acceptable and positive resource for the handicapped child in the family.

Playschemes

The third option available for a family is the playscheme based in one of the residential units where short-term care is given. The playscheme is primarily designed to give the family respite, in addition to short-term care during the long summer holidays. Though the playscheme may appear segregated and special, ordinary facilities are used during the course of the day, for example parks, bars if appropriate, coffee shops, play areas, swimming pools etc. The playscheme is aimed at a priority group: the parents who may have to work during the holidays and/or single parents. The Easter, summer and mid-term school holiday periods and weekends are the times when demand is greatest, hence the development of the playschemes to offer a wider range of options.

Currently playschemes for profoundly retarded and multiply handicapped children have been developed in conjunction with MENCAP and also the integration of suitably handicapped children into ordinary playschemes within the community. One of the basic aims of the playscheme is to replicate the school day and give the child some pleasant experiences and activities during the day in the form of organised play. The playscheme is co-ordinated with the short-term care unit in the family support unit and this combined facility allows approximately 12 children to be cared for at any one time during the Easter and summer holidays. All the schemes together have been found to provide a valuable asset to the supportive families with severely mentally handicapped children.

Case histories

The following case histories are some examples of the successful use of respite care.

Family 'A'

This family comprised husband and wife, older boy and handicapped younger boy, the latter being physically handicapped with a moderately severe degree of mental handicap. The family coped whilst the child was pre-school age and at an assessment centre, but when the news was broken that he had a mental handicap they were distraught and with the help of a caseworker who offered intensive counselling they got through the initial upset and then were in a position to look at the possibility of a period of respite. The child was seen, assessed and introductions were made and the child placed, but during the process other problems were uncovered, such as the mother's reluctance to accept others caring for her child, even though she wanted a break, and the father's non-acceptance of the child's handicap, which manifested itself in working very late hours, avoiding the issues in the home etc. The child's mother was looking for somebody to talk to.

A period of respite helped but initially caused problems in that the void left needed to be filled positively. After intensive counselling, progress was made all round and the support unit was a magnificent outlet for the boy, even though the family had their reservations about its use in the initial stages.

The family now see the unit as their lifeline and the boy plays very well with the other children. Using the unit has been accepted by all concerned and he looks forward to going to the place 'on holiday'.

Family 'B'

This family consisted of two mentally handicapped children both at school, and one non-handicapped boy of school age, in the middle. Family life revolved around the two handicapped children. The family was highly organised and everything had to be done methodically and on time, and because of this constant effort and need to meet deadlines there was a tremendous amount of tension within the household. Both children are profoundly handicapped and the situation was beginning to take its toll on both parents. Again the children were seen, assessed and linked to respite foster parents. This had to be done because of the extent of each one's handicap. This allowed the family time to spend with their non-handicapped child. The two handicapped children are placed at regular intervals with the foster parents: on average a weekend every four weeks and a week to ten days' holiday during the summer. In fact, the family had their first holiday together in 1986. This regular weekend break and some time during the school holidays means that the children are still able to live at home with their family, leading as normal a life as possible, though the pressure is still on the family, simply due to the size of the problem.

This family was first referred in the early days of our scheme and one child was placed initially. The eldest child is now an adult and though respite continued two major hurdles have now to be crossed: the older handicapped person is now reaching adulthood and leaving school, and the family are now worried about post-school facilities for him.

Family 'C'

This family is an Asian family and consists of two handicapped children and two non-handicapped children. Both the handicapped children are attending local schools for children with severe learning difficulties. The family were in desperate need of respite, though for cultural reasons did not want the older daughter to stay overnight, but were happy to allow the younger daughter to stay away from home. Following the usual visits and introductions we were able to provide an overnight stay for the younger child and allow the older child to stay in a particular residential unit from after school to late in the evening, when the family would collect her and take her home. This meant that they were able to have some time with their other children and yet at the same time the handicapped children were able to have different experiences and meet other peers and new social contacts. This arrangement now occurs on a regular basis and is acceptable to all agencies concerned.

In this case too, we discovered language problems as well as difficulties in understanding social work and medical jargon. With the handicapped children away from home the time was used to sort out some of the acute problems, for example using an interpreter and getting a common understanding between the family, medical practitioners, school and the caseworker.

The disadvantages of respite care

The first thing that comes to one's mind is the separation of the child from the family which, if not done positively and constructively, can be very traumatic. One problem that can arise is that an alternative to the family support unit may not be available and parents reluctantly accept the support unit, which in essence could cause more problems than it solves. A child may fret for his or her family and separation can cause emotional and behaviour problems, but we have found if this separation is handled sensitively and positively these difficulties can be overcome.

Conclusions, future trends and some philosophical considerations

Though many local authorities and some health authorities are offering respite care in traditional hostels there is a trend, for good reason, to develop and place handicapped children with respite foster parents for parental relief. Coupled with carers in the community to give relief at home, we see trends that are moving away from regarding people with a mental handicap as being in need of medical services, leading to their admission to the old long-stay hospital or large hostel. Though these developments have occurred, there is still a long way to go and much to do in achieving a comprehensive service for mentally handicapped children and their families. The situation has improved very much, in the sense that handicapped children are not being admitted to the large hospitals and in Manchester this has been avoided for some years now. One way perhaps of ensuring that this continues to provide, as in Manchester, a variety of local services, such as small homes/hostels with four to six beds, respite fostering, family carers, playschemes, sitters, paid staff and volunteers.

The needs of parents also are a very important factor and though at times one may deliberate over who is the client, parent or handicapped person, parents must nevertheless be 'included in the plan' from the beginning. To do this is easier and less harrowing than trying to get the parents interested later if they have not been given their say initially. In some cases in the past, parents had no contact with their child for years and to get them interested is hard work indeed.

Finally, the way forward in serving the handicapped population is to carry out the following:

1. Treat the handicapped person as a person first and handicapped second.
2. Encourage integration at all times where the handicapped person will benefit, not for show purposes.
3. Provide a range of services in small community-based units, i.e., respite fostering, short term care playschemes, appropriate day facilities/opportunities and carers.
4. Work closely with the Health Districts, voluntary organisations and Social Services.
5. Develop appropriate post-19 education facilities particularly for people who are profoundly retarded and mutliply handicapped as the traditional training centre has outlived its original role.

These are just some ideas on ways forward in working with handicapped people. The cost involved is high in terms of finance and staffing but there is one clear factor emerging: mentally handicapped people do not need large institutions to live in, though some may need a form of refuge for a short period of time due to the needs of their particular handicap. If the current models of good practice can be consolidated and further development encouraged, then we will go a long way to meeting the handicapped person's highly individual needs.

Further reading and useful contacts

1. Coupe, J., Porter, J., (eds.) *The Education of Children with Severe Learning Difficulties: Bridging the Gap Between Theory and Practice* (Croom Helm, 1986).

2. Oswin, Maureen, *They Keep Going Away:* A critical study of short-term residential care (The King Edward's Hospital Fund).
3. MENCAP PRMH Project based at Piper Hill School, 200 Yew Tree Lane, Northenden, Manchester – contact person is Loretto Lambe, Tel: 061-998 4161
4. City of Manchester Social Services Department, Respite Fostering Short-Term Care. Contact J. E. Buggy or S. Rowlands, Central Specialists Team, c/o 102 Manchester Road, Chorlton-cum-Hardy, Manchester M21 1PQ. Tel: 061-881 0911
5. Dr Barnardo's Chorley Project – Advice and Information and Sitting Service for Parents of Handicapped People.
   Dr Barnardo's Chorley Project, c/o Dr Barnado's (North West), Divisional Office, 248 Upper Parliament Street, Liverpool L8 7QE. Tel: 051-709 6291/2
6. The City of Leeds Social Services Department (Original Pioneers of Respite Fostering), Merrion House, 110 Merrion Centre, Leeds LS2 8QA. Tel: 0532-463100
7. Exeter Health Authority. The Honeylands Project (Professor F. S. Brindlecombe), c/o Exeter Health Authority, Pintoe Road, Exeter, EX4 88D. Tel: 0392-67171
8. The Spastics Society, Beech Tree House North.
   Further information can be had from them, either Malcolm Jones or Nina Storey at Beech Tree House North, Bamber Bridge, Nr Preston, Lancashire, PR5 8LN. Tel: 0772-323131
9. The Dorset Family Support Services (The Leonard Cheshire Foundation) Family Care Attendant Programme, c/o Dorset Social Services, County Hall, Dorchester, Dorset DT1 1XJ. Tel: 0305-3131

CHAPTER 6

Integration in the mainstream

Dr Seamus Hegarty
Deputy Director, National Foundation for Educational
Research in England and Wales

Most children and young people with severe learning difficulties go to a special school. This is the group traditionally known as the mentally handicapped. Prior to the Education Act 1981, their official designation in Britain was Educationally Subnormal (Severe) [ENS (S)] and most attended ESN (S) schools. With the rejection of the categories of handicap and the static, all-encompassing labels attached to individuals who in reality were very different from each other, the need arose for an alternative way of describing common characteristics. Current preference is for an operational description: the target group is deemed to have in common severe learning difficulties in respect of carrying out certain tasks seen as important by society. Where those of school age are concerned, the tasks relate to educational and, to a lesser extent, social performance. The usage 'severe learning difficulties' may appear vague in comparison with the term ENS(S) with its connotations of specific IQ scores; the latter's precision is however spurious, and it is no great loss in favour of a somewhat more accurate – and less offensive – designation.

The benefits of attending special schools are clear: small classes, expert teachers, adequate numbers of classroom assistants, concentration of specialist resources, ready access to specialist staff such as speech therapists and physiotherapists. Parents can be assured that their child will be in the hands of experts right through their school careers. And when they come to leave school, they will be prepared and counselled by staff who have launched numerous young people with similar difficulties into adult life.

So, why integration? Why should anybody think of dismantling such a valuable form of provision? Or, if not dismantling it, establishing alternative provision with which it must inevitably compete? Why introduce new and untried forms of education just as the existing system is getting established?

It is not such a long time since children with severe learning difficulties were excluded from the school system. Children with severe learning difficulties did not have the right to education in Britain until 1971 (and in Northern Ireland not until 1987). And in some countries, let us not forget, this right is still denied them: the most that many can hope for is physical care, instruction in daily living skills and basic work preparation.

Integration has become an issue for children and young people with special needs over the past 20 years. There were many reasons for this: dissatisfaction with aspects of the special school system, concerns over isolation from peers, worries about the extent to which young people were being prepared adequately for adult life, and a growing conviction that all individuals had the right not to be segregated from the mainstream of society. Debate was fuelled by accounts of practice in other countries, particularly the United States and Scandinavia, by research reports documenting the feasibility of integration and by legislative pressure.

Pupils with severe learning difficulties tended to be ignored in these debates – not because of any lack of goodwill toward them but because they were irrelevant to the basic premise of the debates. Ordinary schools had difficulty enough in providing for pupils with moderate learning difficulties; some, allegedly, were finding the task quite beyond them. Given the extra teaching difficulties presented by pupils with severe learning difficulties, there would be time enough to think about integrating them when ordinary schools were able to cope with pupils who had lesser special needs. Furthermore, much of the debate has been couched in comparative terms, revolving round the respective pros and cons of integrated and segregated schooling. Where pupils with severe learning difficulties are concerned, there has been little integrated provision to draw on. It is not surprising therefore that the debate has not moved very far.

Integration as school reform

There is a more fundamental reason for the lack of progress. Integration has been widely conceived in a limited, static way, and as a result the wrong questions are being asked about it. The comparative focus has led to a concentration on the *location* of education as opposed to its content and delivery. The questions being asked are: Can particular pupils receive as good an education in an ordinary school as they do in a special school? rather than: What conditions must be met for them to receive a good education – in either a special school or an ordinary school?

As a consequence, the debate has been framed in terms of individual pupils and their deficiencies rather than in terms of schools and their failures to provide appropriate teaching. This is unfortunate since it clouds the targets for action. Pupils' failure to learn does not reside simply in themselves. Certainly, there are individual factors relating to sensory impairments, chromosomal disorders and dysfunctions of the central nervous system, which contribute to learning failure. There are environmental factors too: children need appropriate stimulation and learning experiences if they are to develop in normal ways and if these are absent, they are likely to have difficulty in learning at school.

But there are school-specific factors as well. Hegarty (1987) argues that the most pervasive source of children's school difficulties is the schooling system itself. The case is wide-ranging. At a global level, it has to do with the function of schooling in society and the expectations held of schools at different points in time. It has to do also with the set of factors that bear on school effectiveness. Underlying all the different considerations, and giving them a concrete focus in respect of individual pupils, is the curriculum. This is where pupils achieve, and have their achievement acknowledged; it is also where they fail and learn that they have failed.

For present purposes the curriculum can be regarded as a combination of what is taught, the means by which it is taught and the assessment procedures used to monitor learning. When any of these elements is out of step with the learning situation of particular pupils, problems of learning and adjustment can be anticipated. Thus, the traditional subject-based curriculum, with its focus on amassing facts, sets up hierarchies where some pupils will always – and visibly – come bottom. The perceived irrelevance of much of the curriculum to many young people is a powerfully demotivating factor. When this is compounded with teaching methods and assessment procedures that do not mesh with individuals' learning needs, failure to learn and disaffection are likely outcomes.

This argument has most evident force in respect of pupils with moderate learning difficulties and those who exhibit emotional and behavioural difficulties, but it also applies to pupils with severe learning difficulties. The latter may suffer from neurological disorders or other impairments that affect learning, though in practice it can be extremely difficult to specify the link between a given physical or physiological dysfunction and a particular learning difficulty. But such organic limitations do not set predetermined boundaries to pupils' learning. What limits pupils' learning is the nature of the learning environment available to them and how they are taught.

Gunnar Dybwad's well-known dictum is salutary here: 'Because they couldn't learn we naturally didn't teach them. Because we didn't teach them, naturally they didn't learn'. When pupils with severe learning difficulties were deemed ineducable, they did not attend school and academic learning was not even a consideration for them. Now that all are in school, the question is one of the relevance of the teaching provided. Just as their need of expert, closely targetted teaching is if anything greater than that of other pupils, so they have more to lose from inappropriate teaching. If they do not receive imaginative teaching that is carefully matched to their learning situation, they will fail to learn and their organic limitations will indeed become limitations to learning.

This puts the spotlight on schools and the teaching they provide. Integration becomes less a matter of the location of education and more one of its appropriateness. Ordinary schools must ensure that they provide a range of learning experiences geared to the needs of pupils with severe learning difficulties and that they promote their learning to the greatest extent possible. This is the same task as that facing special schools, apart from the crucial fact that it has to be carried out within a different set of constraints and with different opportunities. A comprehensive school cannot organise itself around any one particular group, but must rather provide in a flexible way for pupils with a range of needs. Historically, both primary and secondary schools have excluded pupils with severe learning difficulties from their area of concern – and to that extent none has been truly comprehensive. The requirement of integration is to encompass this new group within a common framework of provision for all pupils.

The challenge to the ordinary school that would cater for pupils with severe learning difficulties is to develop its curriculum offerings and teaching approaches to meet their needs, within the context of the school's entire curriculum provision. The latter is important since otherwise the net effect is to leave pupils with severe learning difficulties still segregated. A special class or department that operates in total isolation from its host school is likely to become a mini special school in all but name. Having neither the independence of autonomous status nor the benefits that should flow from being in an ordinary school setting, it manages to combine the worst of both worlds.

The necessary re-structuring of the curriculum has major implications for the school. Curriculum planning and implementation are themselves whole-school concerns – and indeed provide the central definition of a school – so that curricular provision for pupils with severe learning difficulties cannot be established without affecting curricular provision throughout the school. In addition, any changes must be set within the context of the school's academic organisation since this is the framework within which the curriculum is delivered. Staffing must be considered also, since the kind of staff and the way in which they are deployed determine as much as anything else what changes are possible. At a more general level, factors such as in-service education and the nature and structure of support services are relevant to curriculum change, and will need to be modified if the latter is not to be obstructed.

Some examples

Educating pupils with severe learning difficulties in ordinary schools is clearly a very challenging task. A natural question to ask is: Are there examples of successful practice in schools? Rhetoric and exhortation are all very well but schools must operate in the real world. Unless we can point to schools that are providing an integrated education to pupils with severe learning difficulties, the feasibility of the enterprise has to remain in question.

It is not possible to state how many pupils with severe learning difficulties are being educated in ordinary schools. Official figures from the Department of Education and Science give the national picture but say nothing of what is happening at local level. Also, the figures do not give direct information on the number of pupils being integrated but only on the numbers *not* being integrated, i.e., those in special schools. The national picture is a static one in that the number of pupils with severe learning difficulties in special schools as a proportion of the total age cohort has changed little in the past ten or so years. This picture conceals a certain amount of variation at local level, though it must be acknowledged that information on particular local developments is difficult to come by. There is no evidence to suggest that there is a large number of integration programmes, but there are some. Various published accounts and 'grapevine' information point to the significance of these programmes. While the numbers may be small, pupils with severe learning difficulties *are* being educated successfully in ordinary schools to the general satisfaction of all concerned. This demonstrates that integration is a real option for these pupils: there may be difficulties of practical implementation, but not of principle.

One of the longest-running programmes for pupils with severe learning difficulties in ordinary schools is in South Derbyshire. This dates from the early 1970s when these pupils first became the responsibility of Education. Instead of establishing a new special school, as happened elsewhere, the local education authority established a special centre at an ordinary junior school designed to cater for all children with severe learning difficulties aged two to eleven in the area. (This school already had a centre catering for pupils with moderate learning difficulties.) The centre operated in relative isolation from the rest of the school to begin with, and it took many years for even modest integration to develop.

Secondary provision was established in a neighbouring comprehensive school at about the same time. This was done within the context of a slow learner department catering for about 80 pupils in a school with over 1,100 pupils. About one-fifth of pupils in this department had severe learning difficulties and the rest moderate learning difficulties, although in practice the school does not assign pupils to rigidly defined categories and seeks to blur the distinction between the two groups. In a detailed evaluation of the provision, Hegarty and Pocklington (1982) found that pupils with severe learning difficulties received most of their teaching by means of individual programmes within the department, but they did have access to a wide range of curricular opportunities in the main school. There was a certain amount of integrated teaching; main school staff were positively disposed toward this, though some would have liked more guidance and support. Social interaction between pupils with severe learning difficulties and their peers was unproblematic, if limited in extent.

Another long-running example, though more limited in scope, is provided by the London Borough of Bromley. Its provision for nursery and infant age children with severe learning difficulties has, since the early 1970s, been by means of special classes in ordinary schools. There are five such classes altogether, catering for about 40 children. Staffing is generous: one teacher and two ancillaries plus external support per class of seven to ten pupils. Teaching is mostly within the class but there are some shared activities: music and movement, PE, television, singing, assembly and school events. There is also a good deal of interaction with other pupils. At age eight, the pupils transfer to a special school, usually a school for pupils with severe learning difficulties but sometimes to a school for pupils with moderate learning difficulties.

Kidd (1985) describes an initiative whereby pupils from a special school are transferred, in whole class groups, to a nearby primary school. The pupils have severe learning difficulties and spend most of their time with their own teacher and classroom assistant, but their teaching base is in the middle of an ordinary school and not in a segregated special school. There is in fact some limited academic integration for individual pupils. There is also a great deal of social integration. The development has been well accepted by pupils and staff of the primary school and has been warmly endorsed by parents.

Pupils are now beginning to transfer to a local comprehensive school. This means that pupils with severe learning difficulties in the area will have the possibility of receiving their entire education in ordinary schools. The eventual outcome of this initiative, taken by the special school staff, is that the special school will no longer have any pupils. One of the most remarkable and detailed accounts comes from a parent who describes what was entailed in securing mainstream education for his daughter Samantha (Hulley, 1985). Further information on her experiences of schooling is supplied by Hulley *et al.* (1987) and on classmates' perceptions of her by Swann (1987). Samantha was left with extensive brain damage as well as additional impairments in the wake of infant pneumonia. Her education started at age three in the special care unit of a local school for pupils with severe learning difficulties. Her parents were intent on mainstream education for her, however, and persuaded a sympathetic headteacher to accept her into an infants' school, initially on a part-time basis and after two terms on a full-time basis.

Samantha's education has been highly challenging: 'No-one knew that Sam could work successfully alongside other children until it was tried'. In the event, she made significant progress, especially in communication. All concerned – parents, teachers, specialist staff – are agreed that mainstream education has been successful for her: 'Her life in the classroom is active and purposeful. She is fully accepted as part of her class, and her contact with the other children is a vital part of Sam's life. They benefit as well . . .' (Hulley *et al.*, p.15). At the end of junior school, Samantha transferred to a comprehensive school where it is hoped that she would continue to receive an integrated education.

Links between special schools and ordinary schools

It would be a mistake to see integration as the sole concern of the ordinary school sector. Special schools have an obvious interest in the integration movement since their long-term viability is threatened by it. However, there is another, and potentially more fruitful, interest. This lies in the development of links between special schools and ordinary schools.

Special schools are clearly a major resource in the education of pupils with special needs. Moreover, they will be part of the pattern of provision for some time to come. They are in a position to make a significant contribution to integrated education, since they possess precisely what ordinary schools lack: expertise in dealing with pupils with special needs.

A study at the National Foundation for Educational Research has documented the emergence of links between special schools and ordinary schools (Jowett, Hegarty and Moses, 1988). In 1985, three-quarters of all special schools were involved in a link of some kind with a special school, while a further one-tenth were planning to set up links in the future. The links were extremely varied and could involve pupils, staff and resources, in either direction. Two-thirds of the links encompassed the movement of both staff and pupils. Most pupil movement was from a special school to an ordinary school.

Schools for pupils with severe learning difficulties were particularly active in this respect, with no fewer than 80% of the schools surveyed reporting a current link. A common pattern was for a group of pupils from a special school to be taught by their special school teacher in an integrated session in an ordinary school. In other cases, special school teachers taught classes from the special school in a self-contained way in ordinary schools or advised their ordinary school colleagues on the teaching of pupils with special needs. When pupils did spend time in ordinary schools, they were generally supported by ancillary staff as required.

With a few notable exceptions, the scale of links was modest, with only a relatively small number of pupils and staff involved in any given school. However, this belies their potential significance. Link arrangements rupture schools' existing boundaries. They involve pupils attending a school and teachers working in it where neither group is the responsibility of the headteacher of that school. Clearly, these are interim arrangements and cannot be sustained in the long term. Schools have to face up to the management implications of link arrangements. If they do, and if link arrangements are incorporated into appropriate management structures, the outcome could be a new kind of educational institution that better serves the needs of all pupils including those who have severe learning difficulties.

The way forward

Where do we go from here? We now know that pupils with severe learning difficulties can be educated in ordinary schools, though in practice very few are. Certainly integration is difficult, but there are enough examples of successful practice to show that the difficulties are not insuperable.

There are two possible ways ahead. One is to build on the links between special schools and ordinary schools described above and actually establish the new kinds of institution that they point to. This would be a radical development, but it is a feasible one and well worth considering. The other way ahead is to build up provision in ordinary schools. Mittler and Farrell (1987) put forward an organisational model whereby a local education authority could educate all its pupils with severe learning difficulties in ordinary schools. This is based on shutting existing special schools and establishing units in selected primary and secondary schools (and further education colleges). Senior staff from the special school would have a major responsibility for planning and co-ordinating provision across the different schools and providing leadership and professional support. Staffing would need to be generous in order to provide teaching within the units and support in ordinary classrooms when pupils were being integrated. Pupils would be based within the units but each one would be a candidate for either partial or total integration and would join ordinary classes on an individual basis as appropriate.

Clearly, integration is possible. There are important practical decisions to take on how to move ahead, but the need now is for action, not further deliberation. If we really want to develop integrated provision for pupils with severe learning difficulties, there are well signposted options before us. Either we follow one of these routes, or we settle down to yet more talking about integration, and the year 2000 will see us no further forward than we are today.

Further reading

1. Hegarty, S., *Meeting Special Needs in Ordinary Schools* (London, Cassell, 1987).
2. Hegarty, S., Pocklington, K., *Integration in Action* (Windsor, NFER-Nelson, 1982).
3. Hulley, T., *Samantha Goes to School* (London, Campaign for People with Mental Handicaps, 1985).
4. Hulley, B., Hulley, T., Parsons, G., Madden, S., Swann, W., (1987) 'Samantha', in Booth, T., Swann, W., (eds.) *Including Pupils with Disabilities: curricula for all* (Milton Keynes, Open University Press, 1987).
5. Jowett, S., Hegarty, S., Moses, D., *Joining Forces: a study of links between special and ordinary schools* (Windsor, NFER-Nelson, 1988).
6. Kidd, R., 'Bishopswood Special School: a recent initiative', in Orton, C., (ed.) *Integration in Education: the way forward* (London, Centre for Studies on Integration in Education, 1985).
7. Mittler, P., Farrell, P., 'Can children with severe learning difficulties be educated in ordinary schools?', *European Journal of Special Needs Education*, 2.4 (1987).
8. Swann, W., 'Being with Sam: four children talk about their classmate', in Booth, T., Swann, W., (eds) *Including Pupils with Disabilities: curricula for all* (Milton Keynes, Open University Press, 1987).

CHAPTER 7
Education after school

Fred Heddell
Director of Education, Training and Employment Services,
MENCAP

What will happen when my child leaves school? This question is so
often asked by parents of children with learning difficulties or
mental handicaps. The question highlights a very real concern and
fear about the future, because the days of security and reasonably
well-organised school provision are coming to an end, and the
uncertainties of the adult world are looming large.

After the establishment of a real and proper right to education for
children with mental handicaps in the 1971 Education Act, most
children left school at the age of 16 but went on to the local Adult
Training Centre almost as a matter of course. Some of these centres
did, and still do, provide limited opportunities for a continuation of
the education started in school and some saw their role as developing new opportunities, but the vast majority were based on a light-
industrial workshop-type model.

This lack of choice was a source of considerable frustration for
both parents and teachers, as many felt that young people with
learning difficulties needed further education. Many are just reaching
a point in their lives when they really benefit from formal education
and are likely to make progress way beyond the previously accepted
school leaving age of 16. It was also widely recognised that real
progress is made by people with learning difficulties when they are
given good, well-planned teaching, based on a careful assessment
of needs, for a few hours each day. The normal practice, even in
those ATCs which did provide an educationai programme, is to
provide only a short period each week.

A campaign for the right to full-time education beyond the age
of 16 was therefore mounted in the early 1980s but it was not until
comparatively recently that Education Authorities accepted their
responsibility under the 1944 Education Act to provide continued
education, at least up until the age of 19, for all of the pupils who
required it. The campaign has not yet finished as there are many
people who feel that the statutory right to education should be
extended to at least 21 or even 25 for those who require it.

The growth of further and continued education is therefore fairly new, but it is one of the most exciting and dramatic areas of development in the provision for people with mental handicaps at the present time. Those involved in the field of special education, who have for many years been frustrated by the fact that young people were leaving school just at the point where their rate of learning and development was gaining momentum, are now being given new opportunities to meet the needs. These developments in education after school have been widely welcomed by both parents and professionals who see them as a real and practical example of the way in which the education of people with mental handicaps is at long last being taken seriously.

Options

At the time of writing there are several options open to a young person who is reaching the age of 16 and new ideas are being developed all the time. Under the terms of the 1981 Education Act there should have been a re-assessment of the individual's special educational needs between the ages of 13.6 and 14.6. This assessment should then have been followed by a statement which highlights the needs and suggests the best way to meet them. The options which are likely to be open should include the following:

1. Continuation at school, probably a Special School until the age of 19.
2. Attendance at a College of Further Education on a course specially designed for young people with learning difficulties.
3. A residential course of Further Education and Training for young people with learning difficulties.
4. A place at a Social Education Centre or Adult Training Centre operated by the Local Authority Social Services Department.
5. Link courses with part-time spent in either school or Adult Training Centre and part-time in a local college.
6. Vocational training, possibly through Manpower Services Commission schemes like the Youth Training Scheme.

Before discussing these options in detail it is worth considering, in some depth, the range of needs and the appropriate curriculum structures for each level of training or Further, Continued and Adult Education.

It is now widely accepted that the overall aim for all people with mental handicaps, regardless of their degree of disability, is to develop the skills required to maximise independence within the community at large. For some young people this will mean full vocational training with both job preparation and teaching in the skills that will be required for full residential independence. At the other end of the scale, for young people with profound and multiple handicaps, teaching will probably be heavily biased towards self-care skills like dressing or feeding. Whatever the level of need, the curriculum or training programme should be designed to enable the young person concerned to be as independent as possible, meeting their own needs in all aspects of their lives including their domestic arrangements, their job and, of course, their leisure hours.

The curriculum for full-time Further or Continued Education for people with mental handicaps should therefore contain three main elements as follows:

1. Continued 'academic' instruction with reading, writing and numeracy specifically geared towards developing greater independence in everyday life. This would mean learning to handle money, dealing with weights and measures, basic reading of signs, notices and instructions as well as simple writing. It may also include some of the simple theory needed in vocational training like form-filling, time-keeping or using the telephone. Increasingly this area of the curriculum should also include the use of modern technology like computers or word processors, which may help overcome some of the problems of physical handicaps or even lack of confidence.

   For some young people writing will not be enough and this curriculum area will also need to include continued teaching in speech and communication skills if they are to be able to develop their level of independence.

2. The development of self-care and personal independence skills. This is also a vital curriculum area and would include learning how to use public facilities like shops, public transport, the library or recreational amenities such as the sports centre or cinema. For the less able, the continued development of self-care skills like feeding, dressing and personal hygiene are equally important if any degree of independence or personal dignity is to be achieved. It is also important that careful teaching about relationships at all levels is included. People with mental handicaps often find it difficult to gauge the right level in conversation, becoming over-friendly or over-demanding in social situations and it is vital that they learn about acceptable social behaviour if they are to be fully accepted in the work place or social club. The curriculum should also include carefully balanced teaching about sexual relationships.

3. Opportunities in sport, the arts or even in science or technology subjects should be explored. Some of these experiences may lead onto long-term leisure interests or be of great value in the development of confidence and self-esteem. In others they may only be a passing encounter which none the less broadens

horizons, helps to put other aspects of life into perspective or enriches life generally. This kind of activity is also useful as the basis for a wide range of projects which could be used as methods of developing appropriate work in other areas of the curriculum. A good example would be the reading, writing and numeracy involved in planning expeditions and trips.

Further education in special schools

Many Special Schools have developed separate 'sixth form' units which are designed to provide a more adult environment with new opportunities and, in some cases, a curriculum which is quite different from the rest of the school. This type of provision is usually heavily biased towards the academic curriculum with additional emphasis on the self-care and personal independence skills. As the facilities in most schools are fairly limited, the experiential activities usually have to be provided away from the school site. In recent years some authorities have separated their special schools into primary and secondary so that the young people in the 'sixth form' unit do not spend their whole educational lives at the same school.

Colleges of further and continued education

Views about the most appropriate arrangements for courses in colleges vary, with some operating from existing classroom facilities while others have built special units on the college campus or, in some cases, some distance away. The reason for these variations may well be political rather than operational as there has often been considerable resistance on the part of existing college staff and governors to the establishment of courses of this type. Some feel that a permanent specialist base provides the course with long-term security, while others feel that this approach runs the risk of segregation from the mainstream of the college. The permanent base away from the main college undoubtedly separates the special needs students both in philosophy and practice, but there are good examples of well-integrated courses both with and without special bases in the main college.

The growth in the number of college-based full-time courses over the last few years has been considerable and they are now available in many parts of the country. A major influence on the development of these courses has been the curriculum development work of the Further Education Unit at the Department of Education and Science. Carefully planned and tested curriculum outlines have been published for several different levels of ability and these have had a major influence on the development of courses. One particular reason for this influence may be that a great majority of the staff in Special Further Education are new to the field and need the confidence boost that the FEU packages have been able to provide. One particular package, 'From Coping to Confidence', is a specific staff training scheme which is proving to be both valuable and effective. The FEU is also about to publish a detailed curriculum outline for students with severe learning difficulties. It is based on principles similar to those outlined above and should provide much-needed guidance for staff in this very specialised field.

Adult education

The Adult Education system in Great Britain offers a very wide range of courses and subjects. People with mental handicaps have always been able to take part in these courses in small numbers, but in recent years schemes to encourage greater participation have been developed and there is now a significant growth in the use of these courses.

A great many courses are of a very practical nature and do not require academic skills like reading in order to take part. The most commonly used examples are in the arts, cookery and physical activities but increasingly other courses are being undertaken. For many students difficulties arise in travelling to and from the college or with the social contacts involved and not with the course itself, so to overcome those difficulties a number of befriending schemes have started in different parts of the country. Most of these schemes use a volunteer who would like to undertake the course themselves to act as a friend to the student with mental handicap. In many cases the friends simply travel to and from the college and perhaps take tea breaks together, though in others the friend may act as interpreter or teacher where appropriate. The value of these schemes has now been widely recognised and in some parts of the country, like Inner London, the local authorities have been prepared to employ co-ordinators to link the students and the volunteer friends.

Adult literacy and basic numeracy classes

When the original Adult Literacy Courses were launched in Great Britain in the early 1970s people with mental handicaps were specifically excluded from the provision. The original idea was to try to take the stigma out of illiteracy and stress that there was a very large number of people who had not learned to read and write while they were at school. It quickly became obvious to all concerned that separating people with mental handicaps was extremely difficult, so many Adult Literacy Groups began to make special provision for these people with learning difficulties. The original literacy scheme was also later extended to provide teaching in basic numeracy and other life skills.

The scheme is well co-ordinated by the central Adult Literacy and Basic Skills Unit in London. Classes are run in colleges and schools all over the country, usually as evening classes but increasingly as sessions during the day where this is more convenient. The teaching is in a mixture of group sessions and individual tuition, with the individual work often being done by volunteers. One of the great strengths of the scheme over the years has been the training which has been provided for the teachers and volunteers. A wide range of training material is available and the regular training courses are very popular.

Residential education after school

There are a number of residential colleges which cater for people with learning difficulties. Most are either privately run or run by the voluntary organisations and tend to follow a curriculum which is similar to that which has already been outlined for ordinary Colleges of Continued and Further Education. Most offer courses of either two or three years duration but some offer a course without a fixed length, with students leaving when they have reached a certain stage or standard.

There are many advantages of courses of this type. They offer a greater opportunity for intensive work, particularly in the development of independence and maturity. Many of those involved also feel that there is great advantage for some young people in leaving the family home in the transition between childhood and adulthood and that this in itself helps the student develop.

Those colleges concentrating on the development of independence usually have a progressive programme which starts with supervised care moving on to total residential independence for those that can cope by the end of the course. Good examples of this kind of approach are the training establishments at Lufton Manor, Dilston Hall and Pengwern Hall which are run by MENCAP. Some colleges also offer specific vocational training particularly in areas like agriculture and horticulture, though an increasingly wide range of vocational opportunities are now available. For example, some colleges now provide training in simple motor maintenance, light engineering, building and decorating work and some have shops and cafes as a training base.

For 16–19-year-olds the fees for these residential colleges are usually met by Local Education Authorities, but students over 19 often have considerable difficulty in obtaining financial help. Some students are sponsored by Social Services Departments but the majority have to rely on the Social Security benefits system for financial aid.

Social education and adult training centres

When the majority of young people with mental handicaps leave school either at the age of 16 or 19 they go onto a Social Education Centre (SEC) or an Adult Training Centre (ATC) which is run by the Local Authority Social Services Department. These centres grew out of the Occupation Centres of the 1950s which were created to provide some respite for parents who were reaching the end of their endurance. They traditionally provided occupation through craft activities and gradually moved onto a light-industrial model and by the late 1960s the majority resembled small factories. Many staff as well as parents who were involved quickly recognised that not only was continued education an attractive form of alternative activity but a great many of the trainees made good, rapid progress in the areas which at school had been so difficult. There are many examples of people of 30 or 40 years of age suddenly learning to read or being able to transfer their ability to handle money to other areas of basic numeracy. Towards the end of the 1960s a few enlightened local authorities began to employ qualified teachers to work in their adult centres and many began to include continued academic education as a regular part of the programme. Those centres where qualified teachers were not employed often delegated existing members of staff to develop educational programmes and a basic training in special educational techniques began to be included in the training courses for centre staff.

Unfortunately most centres have limited staff resources with staff ratios between 1:12 and 1:15. This has led to either classes which are too large for real progress, or sessions which are too infrequent for the majority of people with learning difficulties. The usual practice is for groups of five or six students to have an hourly session once, or at best twice, a week. As it is widely accepted that people with learning difficulties make best progress in short sessions each day the situation in most centres is clearly far from ideal.

Fortunately most centres have not restricted their continued education to reading, writing and numeracy. Many have developed a wide-ranging curriculum designed to expand the trainees' ability to function independently in the community at large. There have been some very exciting developments in programmes to teach skills such as shopping, using public amenities, communication, participation in the arts and in leisure activities. One of the most interesting and sometimes controversial areas of development had been the introduction of sex education and training in interpersonal skills. The development of the teaching programmes had been accompanied by a re-examination of attitudes by everybody involved, including parents and often the general public.

The United Nations Declaration, 'The mentally retarded person has the same basic rights as other citizens of the same country and same age', is beginning to be generally accepted and it is recognised that people with mental handicaps need careful and sympathetic teaching in this difficult area because they have a right to sexual activity and many of them will, in fact, exercise this right.

Integration

The principle of integration has been an underlying stimulus in the development of almost all services for people with mental handicaps in the last decade. In some areas of after-school education this has been easily achieved at a superficial locational level with courses in colleges which run alongside mainstream courses. Unfortunately this has rarely led to real functional integration with students working alongside their mainstream peers. In most colleges a degree of social integration has been achieved for the students on the full-time courses by access to the common facilities and this is often assisted by the other students. There have also been some good examples of students with learning difficulties becoming active members of the Students' Union. Unfortunately integration in the sense of shared classroom activity is still rare, though the experience from the Adult Integration project already described shows that this can be a valuable approach for both groups of students. Provision through residential courses is at present entirely segregated, though there seems to be no reason why residential colleges, particularly the polytechnics, cannot provide exciting new opportunities for people with learning difficulties in a similar fashion to those being developed by the other colleges of further education.

Parental involvement

Close links with parents are a traditional feature of all forms of Special Education and many Special Schools take great pride in their home/school links. Parents also have close contact with other services, including the medical authorities and social services provision and they are often well-organised into self-help groups like MENCAP. Indeed, in many cases the actual provision of a service, including the setting up of a school or college course, is the result of the parents' campaigning efforts. Strangely, parents do not as a rule seem to have become closely involved with college-based after-school education. Clearly, for many young people the process of growing up must include a gradual move away from dependency on their parents and this is seen by many as the great advantage of residential post-school education. On the other hand, good special education at all levels depends on very careful planning and this cannot be achieved without the close involvement of the whole family. There is a school of thought which suggests that parents' involvement in post-school education is not helpful, but it is difficult to see how the planning can be undertaken without information from home. Many colleges and other institutions are now beginning to set up parent projects which are designed to help families be involved without being intrusive or over-protective.

Staff training

One of the major needs in the whole field of Special, Further and Continued Education is the development of good staff training. At the moment the majority of staff have been trained in other fields and have adapted their skills to the needs of post-school students with learning difficulties. This means that they may be Special School teachers with no experience of the particular problems of colleges or they may be specialist subject teachers with no previous experience of people with learning difficulties or mental handicaps. For both groups the task can be daunting and special in-service training is required. At present there is no adequate national scheme for this training so teachers still have to rely on their experience, adapting other, not always suitable, courses or using the packages being produced by groups like the FEU or Adult Literacy and Basic Skills Unit.

The future

The developments of recent years have been extremely encouraging but it would be wrong to assume that good educational opportunities for young people with learning difficulties when they leave school are widely available. The availability is still quite limited and varies a great deal in quality. Even though the statutory responsibility for a Local Authority to provide education up to the age of 19 is now accepted, many authorities have only provided the barest minimum and clearly need to use much more imagination in their approach. The colleges which have set up good courses seem to have experienced little real difficulty and there seems to be no reason why others all over the country cannot emulate their initiative. However, very few colleges really see provision for people with learning difficulties as part of their responsibilities and as a result there is a lack of investment in this field. This attitude must be overcome if real progress is to be made.

There is a also a lack of direction and policy both in terms of the actual provision and course content which is inhibiting growth. Variation in courses is obviously valuable but the unco-ordinated development seen at present is causing confusion, with lack of provision in many cases and duplication in others. Clear central guidelines are needed for proper development.

The right to education which continues beyond the age of 19, together with the appropriate financial support, is also a major need which must be recognised by central Government. Somehow the clear message that helping people with learning difficulties take steps, even very small steps, towards their own independence is a good short-term economic investment for long-term gain must be conveyed to those in control of the finance. Hopefully they will see the sense of this and people with learning difficulties will have the same sort of opportunities as the rest of the community.

CHAPTER 8

Work and retirement

Chris Bailey
Manager, Ellingham Employment Resources Ltd

'Hardly ever late' . . . 'Rarely absent' . . . 'Excellent workers' . . . 'Better than some of my normal employees'. These are just some of the comments employers have made about people placed into open employment. People who have undertaken training courses and work experience leading to employment. People with a mental handicap; in some cases, a severe mental handicap.

Contrary to the general belief of both public and professionals, many people with learning difficulties have the potential to success- fully obtain full- or part-time, open or sheltered, socially valued and unsegregated employment.

There are thousands of people with a mental handicap around the country who have been successful in their search for employment. Placements have been secured in a variety of work settings, includ- ing offices, hotels, catering establishments and supermarkets. Jobs range from gardener to office junior, postroom clerk, and general or domestic assistant. The rewards from employment are immense, and in some cases immeasurable. All the training, education and work-related social skills obtained from day centre training pro- grammes come to fruition, enabling the person to participate fully in the very competitive, and sometimes hostile and demanding, world of work. Having a job increases self-esteem, confidence and individuality; the opportunity to work alongside other people increases social awareness and, more importantly, social relation- ships. Work develops the opportunity for integration into, and acceptance by, society itself; the employed person becomes part of our consumer society, and through their experiences they become less dependent on their families and the community and can there- fore take advantage of the social opportunities that surround them. Employment provides a new and exciting dimension to their lives. Work has now become a realistic prospect for clients who have been denied its advantages for so long.

Statutory provision of employment services

Despite the overwhelming evidence that once people with a mental handicap have been given the opportunity of employment they become less dependant upon the day-care services (which all agree are overstretched), very few statutory vocational facilities exist in this country for such people. Some local authorities have promoted vocational opportunities by joint funding projects between Social Services and Health Departments, whilst others prefer to give direct grant aid to voluntary organisations in order that they may initiate and establish such pioneering ventures. Yet more voluntary organisations secure limited term funding through such channels as Urban Aid Scheme or the EEC (European Social Fund).

In the late 1970s, two major and influencial reports were published. Both were critical of the function of day services, highlighting and recommending many areas of change and pointing to a new era of positive development within such establishments. However, local and county authorities have been, on the whole, slow to implement the recommendations made in the survey of 305 ATCs in England and Wales by Whelan and Speake (1977) and in the very comprehensive document from the National Development Group, Pamphlet No. 5 (1977), which encouraged more social development and purpose in day centres than any other work of its time.

Professionals in many parts of the country have argued that now, with such an unstable labour market, day services should plan long-term strategies without the increased risk which independence from day centres might pose to people with mental handicap. Numerous day centres still provide the 'industrial'-type concept in the misconception that employment is no longer a realistic option; therefore little effort is made towards encouraging their clients, who have the potential for work, to continue valuable training and work experience which could eventually enhance their opportunity for an employment placement.

This exploitive type of occupation was highlighted by Norris (1975):

> 'Our attempts to normalise the mentally retarded have declined in the field of industrial contract work. We have a desire to identify ourselves as a community to the mentally handicapped, but unfortunately our attentions reach no further than the work bench.'

For well over two decades this style of day provision has continued, with the opportunities to extend the community resources to the full being at best ignored, and at worst not even known about, by those who advocate for the people they serve. The author has been criticised by many people, including professional colleagues, arguing that to find employment placements for people with a mental handicap today is both unrealistic and totally inappropriate, and that the jobs which are available should be given to the traditional breadwinner. This assumption that a person with a mental handicap does not have the same basic rights as other people is totally unacceptable.

Efforts to provide a variety of different environments in one building has led many to suggest that, as far as training for work is concerned, the day services should define their vocational training programme more clearly and develop a wider use of community contacts. Kings' Fund (1984) stressed:

> 'We are shortly coming to the point where we decide whether we want more traditional day provision or a more community-based service with emphasis on community participation.'

Historically, day centres have relied heavily on fulfilling contractual work. However, the change in the economic climate has now forced companies that previously supplied day centres with contract work to carry out that work themselves. Therefore day centres are having to change their emphasis, in line with the development of care in the community, and move away from the occupational constraints of statutory day-care services towards wider use of integrated adult and further education classes, and public recreation, leisure and community facilities. And of course the provision of work training, on-site work experience and employment is another aspect of this change of emphasis. Many day centres now have a Work Experience Officer, whose role it is to look for opportunities for work experience in and around the community, whilst others have Employment Development Officers who directly negotiate placements with employers. Some of the large employment schemes, such as MENCAP's Pathway and the Shaw Trust, liaise closely with Adult Training/Social Education Centres and imaginative dialogues are resulting in day centres with a new initiative towards vocational training. Work preparation, assessment and vocational choice are key phrases now used in day centres where progressive training strategies are being implemented, with successful results.

Financial payments to clients

Financial remuneration during work training provides a strong motivation to the participants and is an incentive to continue with training to achieve the objective of employment.

At present clients who attend day centres can be given an allowance which invariably does not exceed £5.00 per week. (Some state benefit is lost if payment exceeds this figure.) This disregard payment figure has been increased £1.00 over the previous level by the Social Security Act (1986). However, there is also a higher disregard level of £15.00 for people entitled to the new Disability Premium within the Income Support Scheme (which has replaced Supplementary Benefit). In order to qualify for the Disability Premium, a person must be in receipt of Mobility or Attendance Allowance, Invalidity Benefit or Severe Disablement Allowance.

In some cases clients, with their families, have rejected the opportunity of employment in the fear that certain benefits may not be reallocated should the placement be terminated.

In view of the significant number of projects now emerging in the vocational field, it is very difficult to comprehend how these low levels of payment, even with these new figures, can be reconciled with the client's need to be rewarded for effort, and to have some incentive to remain commited to vocational progress. Both these are important if clients are to realistically obtain a meaningful, valued job and therefore understand the principles of finance and financial responsibility.

For disabled people, and more specifically disabled people (including those with a mental handicap) in employment, the state benefit system is both complicated and confusing. Certainly what is required is a more flexible system which actively encourages that very incentive to work, which is a vital part of the curriculum in a majority of ATCs and similar establishments' work training and experience programmes.

Employment options and vocational choice

What is meant by work? What does work give us in relation to the needs of the community? Initially work provides us with: choice of career; pay; the chance of promotion; the opportunity to work alongside other workers; status; security and social value. All these elements of work should equally apply to the person with a mental handicap in their vocational choice and opportunity. Many local and county authorities are now beginning to recognise that, with careful planning, implementation and training, clients can cross the great divide into employment.

There are many interpretations of the meanings of work and employment. Most people think of employment as a full-time occupation, rather than the choice of options listed below:

1. Full-time/part-time/shift work.
2. Long-term employment.
3. Short-term, temporary work.
4. Seasonal work.
5. Work experience.
6. Job sharing.
7. Sheltered work activities.

8. Work training schemes and courses.
9. Working in a co-operative.
10. Self-employment.

The employment option should include as wide a variety of types of work as practicable and new practices should be initiated within the vocational system. The client's prospects should not remain static and assessment of employment potential should be carried out with a view to realising that potential.

The opportunity for the client to express a vocational choice is very important. Whelan and Reiter (1980) recognised that the concept of choice was an essential part of the training process. They also initiated 'The Illustrated Vocational Inventory', which systematically evaluates a person's vocational interest and knowledge. Some vocational services, and indeed ATCs, use this system as a very good guide on which to base further work training/experience and eventually employment appropriate to the vocational knowledge and interest of the client.

Understanding the client's interest in the work programmes provided by day centres is an area many practitioners are now exploring, along with the client's attitudes, expectations, hopes and anxieties about external work placement. The increase in variety of jobs which Work Experience Officers can now offer is a major new development, arising from interest expressed by clients in particular types of work. To train for a specific job, within the day centres, and progress to work experience, external placement and eventually employment in a chosen area of work has far greater value to the client than an arbitrary placing which may not be relevant to his/her long-term choice.

Family involvement and support

Within the vocational framework there must be provision for the client's family to become involved, and the involvement must not be limited to simply attending reviews, progress meetings and so on. The home environment is certainly the principle learning situation, in which most independency skills are performed or practised (Hegarty, Dean 1984). Therefore, the change in lifestyle not only of the client, but also of the family must be taken into consideration when making the decision to promote a client into an employment placement, or begin training for such a placement. The family must be aware of, and participate in, the planning of the long-term objectives, from the first implication of work training through to the final placing into employment. The family must also be encouraged to take an active and supportive role and feel very much an important part of the negotiating procedure throughout all the stages.

Employment initiatives: the specialist services

With the changing emphasis towards integrated services in day provision, integrated work experience and vocational needs of the clients also have to be met. There is a growing trend for vocational initiatives to be established away from training centre environments. The specialist vocational services should be seen as a complement to existing day services and, together with joint planning, form a comprehensive facility to enhance the vocational needs of clients.

Specialisation, it seems, is the major consequence for initiatives that are now developing from the statutory day provision: projects that are specialised and run on specific vocational lines; staff who are aware of the clients' needs and take into account their respective disabilities and provide a high degree of professional support to the client.

The need for practitioners to know their subject and their clients has never been greater. Staff have to be aware also of changes that may occur in the client's potential and provide a link with the employer. Awareness both of the needs of the employer and the client is of paramount importance. Kings' Fund (1984) stress the point that there is concern because people who know about mental handicap may not be aware of the intricate and complex issues of employment and people who know about employment often know little about mental handicap.

In response to this new individual and developmental approach, new vocational initiatives are being created:

1. In South Wales, the Welsh Initiative for Specialised Employment: a new vocational venture from Swansea was created because of the concern in the present day services in that area. It is supported by the West Glamorgan Common Ownership Development Agency which is primarily involved in workers' co-operatives.
2. In Newcastle-upon-Tyne, provision has been developed into a three tier system. Having been assessed as having potential for work, clients attend the Geoffrey Rhodes Centre where they will be given the opportunity to obtain work experience/ employment after receiving training and support from its staff and services, and being monitored during work placements. The Centre, incidentally, has an Employment Liaison Officer whose role is to encourage local firms and businesses to employ its clients.
3. In East London, Ellingham Employment Resources is totally comprehensive in its approach. It is a purpose-built vocational facility and provides work experience, community work services for the elderly, disabled and housebound, and obtains a

wide range of employment options for its clients, some of whom have severe mental handicap. A very comprehensive back-up and monitoring service ensures that the client achieves his/her vocational potential. The scheme is funded by grants from Urban Aid, EEC European Social Fund (Innovatory Projects) and the local authority (London Borough of Waltham Forest) and is administered by Waltham Forest MENCAP – a voluntary organisation. It is a company limited by guarantee and functions as a company in its own right.

4. In West London, Hammersmith and Fulham has a joint-funded provision called the Blakes Wharf Employment Service. Grants from both the Social Services Department and the Local Health Authority enable Blakes Wharf to seek effective employment placements using the 'key worker' principle, in which an experienced person works on-site with the client to acquaint them more effectively with the job.

5. In Yorkshire, there are a number of people with a mental handicap who are working in a co-operative at the Gillygate Bakery, which started initially as a wholefood shop. It has become so successful that they may expand their services within the next year.

6. Berkshire County Council have Work Experience Officers attached to each of the county's ATCs and have links with various employment agencies and Job Centres.

7. Sheffield have developed a series of 'work stations' where people with varying disabilities can obtain employment appropriate to their individual needs.

8. In Greenock, the Outreach Project was created in 1982 through Urban Aid funding, with the aim of helping people with a mental handicap to integrate into the community and to gain skills which enable them to obtain, and be successful in, employment.

9. Again in South Wales, the National MENCAP Pathway Employment Service, started in 1975, is one of the area's major employment initiatives. The scheme uses a variety of appropriate employment schemes, such as Job Introduction, Sheltered Placement schemes etc., as a means of integrating clients with a mental handicap into employment. Clients are referred to the service through the Disablement Resettlement Officers, ATC managers, careers officers, teachers in further education colleges, social workers etc. A wide range of employment placements have been found for clients with a mental handicap in jobs as domestics, hotel and catering staff, labourers and gardeners, with salaries ranging from £50 to £110 per week.

10. The Shaw Trust, a registered charity and also a company limited by guarantee, started in 1982. It was developed from

three years' funding from the Joseph Rowntree Memorial Trust and other organisations. Its headquarters are at Melksham in Wiltshire, and its Development Officers cover Berkshire, Gloucestershire, Lancashire, Oxfordshire, Wiltshire, Essex and parts of London, Surrey and the West Midlands. The aim of the Shaw Trust is to promote the social and economic integration of severely disabled people into society by using the MSC Sheltered Placement Scheme. Of the disabled and severely disabled people that are placed through the Shaw Trust, about one-third are people with a mental handicap.

11. In the Isle of Wight, there is a comprehensive range of employment and pre-employment opportunities. Based at the Medina Centre in Newport, a diverse range of vocational activities are undertaken and reflect earlier comments regarding community participation. Placements into employment are made using the Sheltered Placement Scheme and the Community Programme. Expansion is planned with the help of a grant from the European Social Fund. To achieve their objectives, therapeutic earnings, Shaw Trust and Community Programme are used to their fullest extent, with a number of new developments to be negotiated to extend further the options available.

It is interesting to note that most of the employment schemes mentioned come from areas where there is high unemployment. All the schemes are effective in their objectives and are placing and supporting people with mental handicaps, some with severe mental handicaps, into jobs in some areas where unemployment stands at 18% or more (a fact which many specialists find difficult to explain satisfactorily).

It is certainly becoming evident through the pioneering work of such national services as MENCAP's Pathway and the Shaw Trust, and local schemes like Ellingham Employment Resources and Blakes Wharf, that the recognition of a person's ability, rather than their disability, now takes precedence and that the concept of care in the community should be complemented by understanding of, and support for, the client's transition towards valued employment.

Employers' reactions

When a client leaves the ATC or specialised vocational service to move into employment, he/she will miss the friends and companionship known for many years. It is unlikely that the person will be able to work for any length of time in a job that does not offer similar opportunities for forming relationships. The employer, in liaison with the ATC or vocational agency, should set a general example, that the client be treated in a friendly, but normal, way. Lowman (1975), a successful employer of people with a mental handicap in his factory, stated:

> 'I would suggest that the dividing line between success and failure in the integration of the mentally handicapped lies essentially in comunication.'

Many employment specialists, negotiating placements with firms, have stated that education of the employer and other employees is often far more important in matters relating to employment of people with mental handicaps than educating the client in the employment placement itself. If a client is to maintain an employment placement, it must offer him/her an effective opportunity to make, develop and maintain social interaction and relationships.

A typical initial reaction of other employees may be one of over-indulgence in treating the client as a form of 'mascot'. This will, naturally, have a detrimental effect on the individual concerned and will develop into an unrealistic and potentially damaging work placement. It is difficult for other workers to see where the line between being friendly and helpful and being over-protective lies. Many employers have noted a great change in people with mental handicaps once they have started work. For example, they adapt to what is considered as more normal forms of behaviour and dress as they begin to feel and become more accepted members of society. Burroughes (1975) noticed a big change in the lifestyle of ex-trainees, now in full-time employment. When they returned to the Centre they displayed their wage packets, their new clothes and bank statements – in fact the 'normal' trappings of our consumer society. Many fears and prejudices from employers and other employees have been, on the whole, based on ignorance of the potential abilities and achievements of clients.

There can be little doubt that financial incentives are a major factor influencing job satisfaction. Some employers, in fact, have commented that increases in pay due to overtime meant far more to the client than other workers.

Government-sponsored employment schemes

Manpower Services Commission (MSC) and its role

The responsibility of the MSC, created under the Employment and Training Act (1973), is to provide the public with employment and training services. It has two major divisions: employment and training. The Employment and Training Act (1973) also legislated that each local authority is obliged to provide vocational guidance and employment placement services under the careers service for young school leavers.

The Department of Employment, in its Code of Good Practice

on the Employment of Disabled People (1984), stated that:

'If disabled people are to receive their full share of opportunities, then it is necessary to increase awareness in the community of the potential of disabled people and of what employers can do to help realise that potential.'

Until recently, however, employers involved in employing disabled people did not consider that the person with a mental handicap could be employable and a valued member of the workforce. The MSC over the last few years has increased its budget to accommodate the growing demand from many agencies such as MENCAP and the Shaw Trust, to initiate new employment schemes with a specific clientele in mind.

The major contact for a person looking for employment is at the Job Centre. It offers a multitude of employment opportunities and often has attached to it the Disablement Resettlement Officer (DRO). The role of the DRO is to have detailed knowledge of local employers and the type of work they are offering and should have close links with, among others, sheltered workshop managers. DROs will be able to offer expertise in vocational guidance, assessment in appropriate training establishments and can arrange MSC financially-aided temporary work placements to gain work experience. They follow up work placements and offer advice on a wide range of provisions offered by the MSC, for example, the possibility of entering an Employment Rehabilitation Centre (ERC) or being placed on the Register of Disabled Persons, both of which could enhance the individual's employment opportunities, as by law firms employing more than 25 people should have registered disabled persons on the workforce (Disabled Persons (Employment) Act 1944). This ruling, however, is under review.

As a continuing development to initiate new ventures for people with disabilities, the Disablement Advisory Service (DAS Team) was created in 1983. Its aim is to provide employers and prospective employers with practical help and advice on how to make comprehensive use of the skills and abilities of people with disabilities as well as a mental handicap, by adopting progressive employment policies and practices.

The advice given to employers can involve job restructuring, provision of special tools and equipment on free loan, and cash grants of up to £6,000 to help with the cost of adapting the workplace. Grants of 75% reimbursement of fares to work are also available for people whose disability prevents them from using public transport to get to work.

Employment Rehabilitation Centres (ERC)

Within the MSC Employment Division, there is the facility for rehabilitation through the ERCs, of which there are 27. Although designed and run for a predominantly disabled clientele, more and more people with a mental handicap use their comprehensive vocational opportunities. According to individual need, courses last on average six to eight weeks, some as long as 26 weeks. Assessment is provided to determine vocational choice and interest. For school-leavers the ERC provides a 13-week Young Person's Work Preparation Course, designed for people with either a mental or physical handicap. The course is intended 'primarily to assist school leavers who because they are physically or mentally handicapped are unlikely to be settled into permanent employment without some form of preparation for the conditions they will meet when entering it' (Whelan and Speake, 1979).

Adult literacy and general workshop experiences are provided with the objective of finding the school leaver employment, or further training. The people involved in attaining these objectives within the ERC are the technical and professional staff, rehabilitation specialists and careers officers.

Job Introduction Scheme (JIS)

This scheme, used by MENCAP's Pathways, enables the Manpower Services Commission to pay the employer who actively engages a client on a trial basis (often six weeks but in some circumstances an extension up to 13 weeks can be granted). It works within the DRO service and it actively encourages employers to take a supportive role by allowing a disabled client the opportunity and the time to pursue a particular job.

Youth Training Scheme (YTS)

Created originally as the Youth Opportunities Scheme, it was renamed and reshaped into the Youth Training Scheme to include a two-year work preparation placement. Under the Equal Opportunities Campaign, many people with a mental handicap who attend special schools are now given the opportunity to take part in the two-year YTS and involve themselves in the full special provisions that are available under the scheme. It provides a foundation of education and training which they need to cope with the demands of a changing labour market.

Sheltered Placement Scheme (SPS)

Undoubtedly this is the fastest growing of special employment schemes. Its purpose is to provide employment opportunities for people with severe disabilities, who can do a useful and valued job of work when given the opportunity to work within their own capabilities. To be eligible, a person must be capable of producing at least 33% of a fit person's output. The clients concerned work the same as the other employees in the workplace, except for the lower output. Many authorities/voluntary organisations are using the SPS as a positive way of achieving employment success for clients who have severe disabilities.

The New Training Programme

The Community Programme, which had a significant success in short-term employment for people with a mental handicap, has now been superceded by the New Training Programme. It is a more detailed training option, with at least 40% of the clients' time now spent on directed training, which colleges, employers or the projects themselves will initiate.

One fundamental change in the new programme is the financial arrangement now in force. 'Trainees', as they will now be called (for all people attending the programme), will receive an allowance of at least £10 more than their benefit allowance. However, certain groups may receive even more.

Practical training is divided into two types:
1. Training with an employer, alongside existing employees.
2. Training on community-based projects.

Further information can be obtained from: 'Training for Employment (PL844 2/88)', Department of Employment, Caxton House, Tothill Street, London SW1H 9NF.

Asset Centres (Assistance Towards Employment)

Asset is a relatively new initiative to encourage the disabled to find or keep a job. There are at present three Asset Centres throughout the country at Wrexham, Gillingham and East Ham, London. The scheme gives clients the opportunity to prove to themselves and to potential employers that they can make a positive contribution to work. Areas covered at an Asset Centre are training in the development of specific skills needed to obtain work, 'on site' work experience and vocational assessment. Benefits are not affected by attending Asset, though Asset will also pay a weekly allowance for longer term attendance (more than two weeks) and subsequent work experience placement. Referrals are through the Job Centre provision, through the DRO service.

Any further detailed information on any of the above work/employment schemes can be obtained from the local DRO based at the Job Centre.

Retirement

Due to the increased success in medical technology and, more specifically, better diagnosis and treatment of diseases which would have been fatal for many people with a mental handicap in the past, it is now well accepted that such people have a normal life expectancy.

This in turn has led to increasing concern over the provision of facilities which meet the changing needs of the elderly person with a mental handicap.

Many people coming to the end of their working life reassess their recreational and leisure opportunities in line with their new life-style. People who have been employed for many years are often given courses on retirement by their firms and companies, covering such topics as use of one's leisure time, saving and investing wisely, pension and benefit rights and making and maintaining friends in a new environment. Local authorities now recognise the importance of providing a wide range of recreational provision for this age group. Recreation and leisure centres offer their extensive and rapidly-expanding facilities at reduced, affordable prices, therefore increasing the range of opportunities for older people to participate. Drop-in Centres, which use occupational work facilities to encourage those who feel they still want to contribute in some measure to an industrial environment, in a social atmosphere, are one type of facility which is developing as a result of demand. Social clubs run specifically for retired people also fulfil a need for clients. Luncheon clubs help people make new friends and adult education classes offer recreational sessions for people of retirement age and beyond, with courses which encourage the learning of new skills and crafts; however, some areas around the country offer sparse facilities and should start to develop a growing range of services for this clientele.

Retirement from day centres

There is no 'official' retirement policy for clients attending Adult Training Centres or similar establishments, and often they attend until such time when age, illness or frailty means that the day centres can no longer provide the type of care they may need.

Within the day centres there is a wider appreciation of this emerging clientele which cannot be catered for adequately within the ATC environment. Many operate a token policy of retirement, or re-adjustment, to encourage more active use of community facilities appropriate to the client's particular needs. It is a well-known fact that many people with a mental handicap who have reached retirement age and who are introduced to the ordinary social clubs for the elderly integrate well, and often participate in the social life more fully than other club members.

Clients' attendance at such provision can only be achieved with the support of the day services. Staff should therefore actively pursue these activities so that those with the necessary social skills are able to integrate more effectively. This in turn develops a greater opportunity for making relationships outside the sheltered environment of the Adult Training Centre. There are some good examples of this sort of development around the country. In Birmingham, provision is made specifically for people who are becoming of an age when day-centre provision is no longer appropriate. In Waltham Forest, an 'Over 50s' provision has been created to encourage more people with a mental handicap to participate in a variety of social and leisure opportunities outside the ATC. There are also a growing number of day centres which now provide their own social club. This is in response to the growing need of older people attending day centres who, because of the severity of their disability, find it increasingly difficult to interact with the younger, more able, clientele. More comprehensive provision needs to be made available for this group.

Throughout the whole of a client's training and education, it should be recognised that the client will eventually retire from the day centre, so that their retirement is properly planned and an effective relocation (if and where possible) to more appropriate environments can be implemented. The 'retirement' age for people attending day centres can vary dramatically. In some instances, the client nearing 55 may not feel their age and may not wish to take an active part in the retirement plan offered. On the other hand someone of the same age or younger may be showing signs of tiredness, reduced mobility and so on and may benefit from such a plan. The fact that clients are offered the opportunity to experience the option, whether or not they wish to participate, leaves the choice with each individual. It must be remembered, however, that if a person has attended the ATC for many years it may well be the centre of that individual's life – with friends and interests all in this one place. Attendance at the day centre should therefore not cease suddenly and totally. Gentle transition should be encouraged, to help the person make the change in life-style, if appropriate, and of benefit to that person.

The approach to the subject of retirement from day centres must be treated with sensitivity and based on the individual needs of each client. Retirement should be valued not only by the client but also by staff and practitioners.

Retirement from work

Retirement from work for the person with a mental handicap is an area which has rarely, if ever, been discussed, primarily because many people with a mental handicap have not been employed regularly for most of their lives.

For the person with a mental handicap who has worked up to the legal age of retirement they should expect the same facilities and support which other employees receive. As already mentioned, many companies provide very comprehensive opportunities to equip their workers nearing retirement age with practical skills. For the person with a mental handicap, such opportunities could be offered either solely by the company, or with the support of the day or specialist vocational services, if required by the client.

Some specialist vocational services actually co-ordinate their own post-retirement plan based on local knowledge of resources available to people with a mental handicap. Attendance is offered to clients attending ATCs. The principle objectives for retirement should be identical to those of employment, and should take into account the client's increasing needs as they get older. A good retirement option should fulfil the following:

1. Support the client.
2. Have purpose.
3. Be valued by the client.
4. Provide a changing and supportive structure for their new life-style.
5. Be active and meaningful.
6. Prepare the client for full and constructive use of their time.
7. Increase the client's quality of life and integrate as much as possible to achieve that purpose.

If retirement for people with mental handicaps is to be viewed as a realistic contribution to care in the community, then day centres, specialist vocational services and the public sector have to be aware that the options available to the community as a whole must include opportunities for people with mental handicaps to integrate more actively at retirement and post-retirement age.

Further reading

1. Burroughes, *Placement of ATC Trainees into Open Employment*, a report of the proceedings of a two-day conference held at Kings' Fund Centre (Kings' Fund Centre, 1975).
2. Hegarty, S., Dean, A., *Learning for Independence* (Further Education Unit, Stanmore, Middlesex, 1984).
3. Kings' Fund Project Paper No. 50 *An Ordinary Working Life* (King Edward's Hospital Fund for London, 1984).
4. Lowman (1975) 'Permanent Employment in Industry for the Mentally Handicapped Person' from Elliott, J., Whelan, E., (eds.) *Employment of Mentally Handicapped People*, a report of the proceedings of a two-day conference held at Kings' Fund Centre, London (Kings' Fund Centre, 1974).
5. Manpower Services Commission *Code of Good Practice on the Employment of Disabled People* (Sheffield MSC, 1984).
6. National Development Group Pamphlet No. 5 *Day Services for Mentally Handicapped Adults* (National Development Group for the Mentally Handicapped, 1977).

7. Norris, D., Chapter XII 'Special Education and Training' from Kirman, B., Bicknell, J., (eds.) *Mental Handicap* (London, Churchill Livingstone, 1975).
8. Whelan, E., Reiter, S., *Illustrated Vocational Inventory* (Manchester Copewell, 1980).
    Whelan, E., Speake, B., *Adult Training Centres in England and Wales: Report on First National Survey* (National Association of Teachers of the Mentally Handicapped, Manchester, Revel & George, 1979).
9. Employment & Training Act (1973) (London, HMSO).
10. Disabled Persons (Employment) Act (1944) (London, HMSO).
11. Social Security Act (1986) (London, HMSO).

CHAPTER 9

Options in day service provision

James Cummings
*Formerly Director of Education, Training and Employment,
MENCAP*

No neat recipes for options which should be open to people with
mental handicap can be offered. There have been suggestions that a
single Department of the Handicapped would ensure greater equity
of provision and more flexibility of choice. Most workers in the
fields of mental handicap reject this, believing that such a move
would lead to further segregation, rather than integration. The
writer shares this view and accepts that the way forward to providing greater choice can only come through extended and intensive
co-operation of various local authority departments, voluntary and
community agencies and the widened interest of the general public.
Social Services Departments must enlist the co-operation of the
Local Education Department, the Leisure and Community Services,
the Community Mental Handicap Team, and any other statutory
providers of day services.

The first and essential stage in providing maximum choice of
optional activities is a recognition that whilst the Social Services
Department has a duty to make special provision this does not in
any way absolve other service departments from providing for
people with mental handicap. A disability does not make anyone
less of a citizen and should not affect their entitlement to a share of
ordinary services.

Unless this first step takes place it is unlikely that more ambitious
efforts will follow. Some Adult Training Centres have already
launched 'out-reach' activities with the co-operation of community
organisations. The process of creating resource centres and widening the experiences of people with handicaps has started but, it
must be admitted, in only a small way. Does the will exist to
vitalise the approximately 500 Adult Training Centres and give a
more stimulating life to the 50,000 people attending them? This
number may double by the end of the century; we cannot wait for
radical and comprehensive change: we must begin now, step by
step. There is no magic or mystical formula existing or needed. No

new knowledge or innovative thinking is required – a vast and illuminative literature already exists. What is required is increased action in providing activities of a kind which are relevant to the individual and changing needs of people with mental handicap.

This chapter consequently has no high ambition, but examines some of the thinking, ideas and practices which may open up possibilities for people with handicaps.

Day service responsibility

Social Services Departments are at present the main providers of day services for adults with mental handicap. They derive this duty through various schedules of the National Health Service Act 1977. Schedule 8, paragraph 2, of the Act details various provisions that include 'the provision for persons whose care is undertaken with a view to preventing them from becoming ill, persons suffering from illness and persons who have been so suffering, *of centres or other facilities for training them or keeping them suitably occupied* and the equipment and maintenance of such centres'.

In specifying 'centres' as one way of meeting the needs of mentally handicapped people the Act endorsed a type of provision with a considerable history behind it. By viewing mental handicap as an illness, a controversial point was raised which is still unresolved and beyond the subject matter of this chapter. It will also be noted that 'other facilities' may be utilised and a number of authorities provide generic centres which accommodate people with a variety of handicapping conditions. Whilst this is understandable from a financial and staff resource point of view, it emphasises segregation with its consequent effects. The number of local authorities using this type of day centre is relatively small and, to the writer's knowledge, little attempt has been made to justify it by evaluative evidence. Adult Training Centres (ATCs) and Social Education Centres (SECs) succeeded the Occupation Centres pioneered by a number of voluntary bodies, and some local authorities, after World War I. They were an alternative preferable to institutional care, but were still a variation of segregation and, despite developments, have largely remained so.

The concept of the day centre was therefore not a creation of the 1977 National Health Service Act, but an inheritance from earlier legislative enactments which were restrictive and often punitive in origin. Activities within occupation centres were rooted in the concept of ineducability and at best provided 'training' programmes of a varied nature. The writer is certainly not alone in having recollections of an ancient church hall in which simple woodwork and weaving were the activity of the more able, whilst the less able sorted strands of coloured wool into matched heaps which at the end of the day were put back in a sack. Had there been an attempt to evaluate any skills learned, this task would have had a point, but there was no such attempt. This was not atypical but the anecdote serves a purpose; it highlights the fact that despite undoubted progress made in a few decades, *we have so far failed to devise a system of day service provision which provides for each mentally handicapped person the right activity according to his/her needs at a particular time and stage of development.*

By the passing of the 1970 Education (Handicapped Children) Act, the stigma of ineducability was removed and children have benefited from the considerable new thinking and improved educational provision resulting from this Act. It is paradoxical that the very children who benefited most from admission to educational provision find that on completion of schooling at 16 or 18 years of age, the best they can hope for is a place in an Adult Training Centre, which may be for life. If fortunate they may find that they are in a centre where management are aware of new ideas and are striving to provide activities which widen and enlarge personal experience. They are more likely to find themselves in an ATC which holds a traditional view that its job is to provide occupation from nine o'clock to four o'clock.

A major weakness hindering the delivery of a comprehensive day service providing optional activities is the lack of a national policy on day services for people with mental handicap. A consortium of organisations in 1986 ('Count me in for Community Care') called for 'a central Government inter-departmental liaison committee, drawing its membership from Ministers in Health and Social Services, Environment, Education, and Transport departments, to be established. This committee should publish an annual report on community care and submit it to Parliament'. This call, which came jointly from Dr Barnardo's, Mind, The Spastics Society, and MENCAP, has elicited no response. It is difficult to see the logic of calls from central Government to local authorities to increase joint planning provision and co-ordination, whilst showing such reluctance to give a lead.

Advocating a more individual approach to day service provision for mentally handicapped people entails considerable optimism. Social Services Departments are under pressure to extend services, yet they are under-funded and consequently under-staffed. Discharges from mental handicap and psychiatric hospitals mean that additional day care has to be provided, which often results in prospective clients in domiciliary care going on waiting lists. There is little real knowledge of community care provided relative to needs, and such care as exists is rarely subject to monitoring and evaluation. Increased family breakdown and problems raised by the care needs of an ageing population challenge the expertise and imagination of the most experienced director of social services.

Realism might suggest that this is not the right time to advocate an up-grading of day services for mentally handicapped people – but then there never has been a right time for demanding priority for them. For this reason parents and friends of mentally handi-capped people must do everything to ensure that their needs are well represented in priority terms. Campaigning is a legitimate manner of influencing and informing local and national policy makers about the needs of handicapped people. Ideas will only be made real through public pressure and a greater extension of public education relating to the needs of mentally handicapped people.

Changed concepts relating to day services

Three main concepts have emerged relating to day service pro-vision in recent years altering our perception of the needs of people with mental handicap. They are as follows:

1. The normalisation principle.
2. Social integration.
3. The provision of community care.

The concepts are obviously inter-related and underpinned by the recognition that handicapped people have 'rights'. Such rights embrace legal rights established by the laws of the land, and human rights evolved in a free society and based on philosophical and humanistic ideas about the nature of man and his efforts to establish equitable and reciprocal relationships within society. Whilst it is true that rights must be related to responsibility, people with mental handicaps have for too long been deprived of both human and legal rights. Recent decades have brought a realisation that most people with mental handicap can accept the responsibility which accompanies these rights, although in some cases support may be needed. The conviction that people with mental handicap have rights is an obvious pre-requisite for the operation of com-munity and social integration programmes.

The normalisation principle

The normalisation principle has had a strong influence in the past decade. Bengt Nirje, one of the originators of the principle, ('The Normalisation Principle and its Human Management Implications' in *Changing Patterns in Residential Care*, President's Committee on Mental Retardation, Washington, 1969) defines it as 'making available to the mentally handicapped, patterns and conditions of everyday life which are as close as possible to the norms and patterns of the mainstream of society'. Despite the existence of considerable literature on the subject there is a wide variation on how the principle is applied. This is not surprising in view of the temptation to over simplify the interpretation of the principle.

To provide a physical and structural environment which encourages normal patterns of life is not difficult, given initiative and imagination. Moving towards normalisation of social interaction is more challenging, given the wide variations in handicapping conditions. The person who is free from any physical impairment and whose learning disability is mild will obviously find it easier to conform to 'patterns and conditions of everyday life' than someone with multiple physical handicaps and profound retardation. When treated in a more normal way by the general public, people with mental handicaps will, in most cases, react relatively normally. This is not to deny that some people with mental handicap may exhibit idiosyncratic behaviour of a certain type. A mentally handicapped person may be able to travel on a bus, pay the fare and find the way safely despite a speech problem. If he or she is a particularly garrulous person, the speech difficulty will not prevent him or her trying to make conversation. Fellow passengers may find this embarrassing, but it is interesting to note the ever-increasing acceptance by the public of mentally handicapped people on public transport.

The normalisation principle is no panacea and staff and clients have to work hard testing out its boundaries in everyday life. Developing social skills and widening experience have to include some understanding of behaviour and attitudes and how to react in a wide variety of social situations.

The Individual Programme Plan (IPP)

The IPP is a practical plan through which the normalisation principle can be advanced. The IPP aims to identify in some detail the strength and weaknesses of the handicapped person, to assess his/her positive characteristics, interests, aspirations and current ability. Central to the IPP is the participation of the client and his expressed wishes, which are as far as possible reflected in the personal programme.

Though the IPP makes considerable demands on staff, for the client the emphasis on individualism provides a counter balance to the more usual group activities. The succes of the IPP depends on systematic planning, based on the full involvement of the client, his/her family and all agencies who provide, or might be able to provide, suitable services and support. An IPP should be based on a written statement which includes present performance and defines future goals, and sets out an objective evaluation system of progress and achievement. Whilst the planning of the IPP will result from teamwork, there must be one person whose responsibility it is to ensure that the agreed plan is implemented and monitored.

The operation of an IPP should be seen as the appropriate basis for ensuring a service designed to meet the individual needs of the client. The organisation of all available community resources should be fully explored in order to provide the support needed to enable the handicapped person to move towards ever-increased independence and integration in the community. This may well include the use of community organisations, and other resources at present not within the purview of mental handicap services.

Readers are referred to *Individual Plans for Mentally Handicapped People* by R. Blunden, Mental Handicap in Wales Applied Research Unit, Ely Hospital, Cardiff, for fuller information.

Day service delivery and choice

The opportunity to make choices is something new in the life of many mentally handicapped people. After all, it is not so long ago that the most simple choice was denied them, particularly if they were hospitalised. It is now generally accepted that mentally handicapped people have a right to be consulted and given choice as far as possible. Self-advocacy groups of handicapped people are being much more assertive about their needs and preferences. A particular benefit of self-advocacy is that these more able people can effectively speak, not only for themselves, but also for their less able fellows.

There is a current fashion to generalise about freedom of choice for people with mental handicap as though all share equal capacity for exercising choice. To deprive choice to anyone who can exercise it is demeaning and unjustifiable. But acknowledgement of possible limitations in some people is no denial of their human dignity; it is a recognition of our responsibility. We have preferred to use the term mental handicap rather than special educational needs. The ability to exercise and handle choice effectively is governed by the degree of intellectual, emotional, physical and cognitive development of the individual. For this reason the traditional terminology has been used in the belief that it is more useful in delineating the needs and problems of the individuals to whom this paper relates. This is, of course, a contentious issue, but pejorative labels result from people's thinking, not from the label itself.

It is deceptively easy to theorise about choice and to overlook the complex issues of volition which govern choice. The point has been made that personal development of the handicapped individual is the goal towards which we strive. We find it difficult to have a valid concept of personal human development which does not include some degree of choice for the individual. It is equally true that as choice is volitional it is dependant on many other characteristics of personal development which begin in infancy and in some respects continue throughout life. This paper is concerned with day services in adolescence and adulthood but it is axiomatic that the efficient and effective utilisation of day service provision will be dependent, to a great extent, on early childhood training, education and consequent development.

A changing role for the ATC/SEC

It is generally accepted that the role of the Adult Training Centre or Social Education Centre is changing. There is limited knowledge about the degree and extent of such change, largely due to the nature of local responsibility for the delivery of such services. There is an urgent need for a new national survey and a much greater degree of support from central Government to meet the extended role of community care. Despite the confused and varied nature of day service provision there is considerable evidence that some authorities are endeavouring to operate more individualised services and provide options for personal activities based on various versions of the IPP and the concept of normalistion.

More Social Services Departments are moving towards the extended use of community resources such as swimming pools, sports centres, youth hostels, drama and dance projects and 'drop in' centres. Student councils and self-advocacy groups are increasingly to be found in Social Education Centres and contribute to a more imaginative use of resources. (*Advocacy: The UK and American Experience*, Sand and O'Brien, Kings' Fund Paper 51.)

The arts and mental handicap

It is noticeable that development in the arts field has been much less rapid than in the field of sport and recreation. There exists a United Kingdom Sports Association for People with Mental Handicap co-ordinating such activities but nothing similar exists to co-ordinate the creative arts, despite recommendations made in the Attenborough Committee's Report on Arts and Disabled People and in MENCAP's Report of the *Ad Hoc* Leisure Committee. (See 'Further reading' at the end of this chapter.)

The value of the creative arts in expanding self-expression and aiding concentration and emotional development cannot be over emphasised. They have a supreme advantage in bringing about individual satisfaction through group interaction. Drama and theatrical productions in particular present possibilities for using a variety of talents and skills such as costume making, scenery construction, back-stage work and programme selling. They also provide the possibility of assimilating family, friends and other non-handicapped people, thereby encouraging integration.

Multi-media presentation is more associated in our minds with up-market art galleries than with mental handicap. Yet it provides exciting opportunities to incorporate painting, paper sculpture, lighting, sound effects and movement. The Lung Hu Theatre

Company in Edinburgh are probably the most experienced and adventurous in demonstrating the value of multi-media presentation for mentally handicapped people.

Their most recent production 'Light up the Land' produced in collaboration with the Slide Workshop has had an enthusiastic reception. *The Scotsman* (9 November 1987) describes how a combination of acetate, felt pens, coloured ink, sculptured sand, polythene material, sound and projection have resulted in showing 'how simple techniques can emerge in a flood of beauty, especially satisfying for those whose capacity to create has hitherto seemed limited'. The theme of the performance has resulted from visits to beach, woodlands, scrap yards; bonfires and other experiences have fed and stimulated the imagination of the participants. The Lung Hu Theatre Company is fortunate in having committed professionals associated with it, particularly as they are demonstrating that creativity is nurtured through encouraging initiatives rather than imposing ideas and standards. The Lung Hu Theatre Company took its name from their performance in Edinburgh three years ago of the Chinese tale 'Lung Hu's Monkey'. Their continued exploration of new ideas which lend themselves to community integration is a valuable contribution in extending optional activities for handicapped people.

The expanding arts provision for mentally handicapped people can be seen through a perusal of the Arts Council Directory, *Art and Disability Organisations and Projects*. Apart from the projects listed involving mentally handicapped people there are many others with integration objectives. Staff who very often work in relative isolation are surprised to discover how many more colleagues exist. Despite the expanding activity in this field we touch only the fringes of the needs and possibilities.

Sports and physical recreation

Since the Special Olympic movement was founded in the USA by Eunice Kennedy Shriver (1968) the movement has become world wide. The first games for mentally handicapped athletes were held in 1968; the UK Special Olympics was formed in 1979 and has now more than 60 groups with more being formed. The UK Sports Association for people with Mental Handicap set up in 1980 co-ordinates the interests of 26 organisations. The constituent members include Associations of County Councils, Metropolitan and District Councils as well as representatives of many organisations concerned with the promotion of sports and physical recreation. In extending a variety of optional activities to handicapped people in the realm of sports there is a great advantage in the fact that sports people seem to respond readily to the challenge of sharing their activities with handicapped people.

Whether it is angling or archery, sailing or snooker, cycling or cricket, co-operation and help in coaching and participation in events has resulted in a new sense of accomplishment for many mentally handicapped people. Their success in sports brings increased self-esteem and promotes social integration.

Towards transition

The transition towards a fully comprehensive day service will be gradual. There must be a recognition that any precipitous move to dismantle Adult Training Centres could be disastrous. The point has been made that the titles of ATC and SEC have little real significance. There are ATCs and SECs which have gone a long way towards widening activities and initiatives in such a way that they could be appropriately described as Resource Centres. The activities described by Tinto in the report 'Development of day services in statutory strategy' in *Working, Learning and Leisure* (MENCAP South West Region, 1987) relating to West Devon Social Services are typical of progressive and imaginative authorities. A working party consisting of day centre managers, a social worker, a community worker, a psychologist and a community nurse have produced a draft document defining the role of day centres in more precise terms than is usual. The question of assessments, IPPs, community programmes and education were discussed and will form the basis of a redefined role of Adult Training Centres for the authority.

There is a considerable ferment of activity country-wide, but greater exchange of experiences and cross-fertilisation of ideas is needed. Failing the assumption of responsibility by a central Government department (an unlikely and possibly undesirable alternative) there has to be more efficient and effective ways of utilising joint planning and funding mechanisms. A day service which aims to extend options to clients within the widening needs of care in the community can do so only by a system of shared responsibility. The needs of many mentally handicapped people will require continuous provision throughout life. *Day Services – Today and Tomorrow* (Chapter 5) has outlined a systematic approach to the reorganisation of services and resources. The ideas are not original, in fact much was culled from submission by social service providers, but they do provide an adaptable framework for a more systematic approach than prevails in many authorities at present.

Choice and risk

It will be clear that the writer of this chapter views the nature of choice as emerging from concomitant aspects of personality developments. The way people (with or without handicaps) exercise choice is subject to highly idiosyncratic factors. The influence of relatives, friends, teachers, films, television etc. may play a part in extending aspirations and possibly choices. The reasons for entering into activities and indeed for choosing certain relationships may be difficult to define, even for the person making the choice. This is true for all of us, but has special significance for people with mental handicap. Activities naturally centre round people and, as has been mentioned, relate to community integration and interaction. The move from institutional life to community living is liberating but not without risks. The vulnerability of some mentally handicapped people in an increasingly hostile inner-city environment cannot be ignored. We have touched on the absolute necessity of support, part of which must be counselling, advising, and providing information which helps minimise the risks to which we are all subject.

The objective of community living is to enable handicapped people to have more control of their own lives but we do them no service if we fail to provide the guidance and information which will enable them to live in relative safety. The individualised plan has been commended as it enables people to accept that freedom of choice is not absolute but is conditional on wise selections of options which are realistic and appropriate.

Parents and families of people with a mental handicap are very often more than nervous about the freedom of movement afforded to people living in unstaffed homes and hostels. We have a duty to recognise the often legitimate basis of their fears and to ensure that extended options in life-styles are as far as possible related to the capacity of the handicapped person to cope with them. In our eagerness to extend options, we must always be aware of the fact that mental handicap is variable and, unless the phrase is meaningless, will in some cases impose limitations. This in no sense dehumanises the mentally handicapped person any more than accepting that blindness, paralysis, deafness or other physical disability is part of the human condition. Our recognition of the value of all human beings must be based on deep perceptions rather than the possibility of personal accomplishments.

Profound handicap

It would be remiss if we failed to emphasise the necessity of endeavouring to provide appropriate options to profoundly and multiply handicapped people. There is an inclination to ignore simple preferences on their part. Such preferences are often expressed in gesture where speech is limited or undeveloped. In special care units even the most devoted staff put people out in the sun in groups because 'it's good for them' despite the fact that grimaces and head-turning indicate that in some cases a place in the shade would be preferred. Both children and adults are frequently fed by staff in the interest of tidy feeding when the acceptance that a rather messier mode of self-feeding could be more productive in the long run. This is not meant to minimise the difficulties facing the dedicated staff who serve the needs of profoundly and multiply handicapped people. However, an extension of professional training could assist staff to detect and identify the subtle nuances of reactions through which multiply handicapped people may signify preferences.

If we refuse to acknowledge profoundly handicapped people's preferences we are in danger of denying all mentally handicapped people the dignity which even limited choice can afford them. Our present preoccupation with choice is based on the realisation that development is further retarded and personality stunted when choice is denied to any individual.

Summary

This chapter is reflective rather than dogmatic. A theoretical list of optional activities would have been easy to construct but of doubtful value. We have chosen to consider how the capacity for meaningful choice may be developed within contemporary concepts of service provision. Professional and imaginative staff should not find it difficult to conceive and provide optional activity but this will be of limited value unless the client has developed a capacity to express and exercise preference. The social and educational infrastructure relating to personal development has been touched on and the difficulties in the variable nature of mental handicap recognised.

The limits of choice for some mentally handicapped people have been recognised but the need for sensitively and experimentally stretching such limits emphasised. Whilst advocating the necessity for a transformation of Adult Training Centres, we have recognised the value attached to them in the present circumstances. The extended provision of care in the community presents challenges of choice not only to clients but to service planners and providers. If we fail to make wise choices we could well substitute institutional care by even poorer community care.

Providing a service meeting the ever-changing needs of handicapped people will depend on the value which we accord them as fellow human beings.

Further reading and useful contacts

1. Royal Society for Mentally Handicapped Children and Adults (MENCAP), 123 Golden Lane, London EC1Y 0RT.
2. *The Arts and Disabled People* (The Arts Council).
3. Report of the *Ad Hoc* Leisure Committee to MENCAP.
4. MENCAP (South West Region), 17 High Street, Taunton, Somerset.
5. *Day Services Today and Tomorrow* (MENCAP).

Personal relationships and personal fulfilment

Ann Brechin
Lecturer, Health and Social Welfare Department, Open University

'If we love or are fascinated or are profoundly interested, we are less tempted to interfere, to control, to change, to improve. My finding is that, that which you love, you are prepared to leave alone.' Maslow (1973) p.18.

This provocative quote is intended to set the agenda for this chapter. If it is true, what does it mean in practice for the personal relationships and personal fulfilment of people with learning difficulties? Does it imply a tolerance verging on neglect, an ideal world in which love makes no demands, or does it simply serve to make us question our unthinking reliance on interventionist approaches?

In contrast to Maslow's observation the reality is rather different. We have become, in our society, rather good at teaching people what they ought to do, how they ought to behave, what they should strive to become. We do it to our children, to our pupils in school, to our mass media audiences, to our husbands and wives, and no less, to particular groups like people with learning difficulties. Maslow calls this process 'extrinsic learning' and sees our tendency to make decisions about other people's needs reflected in our continual attempts to push people into particular predetermined moulds. In his quotation he conveys an alternative vision of the world, of human relationships; a world in which 'intrinsic learning' can be encouraged by a different kind of relationship, one where the individual comes to his/her own view of what needs to happen. 'Intrinsic learning' he defines as 'the process of growing into the best human being one can be'.

He is not alone in pointing to such distinctions in approach. Carl Rogers' influential approach to counselling and psychotherapy (Rogers 1951, 1961) is built upon the same underlying commitment to total acceptance of each individual as they are, as the starting point for any process of growth. He sees people as drawing strength from a genuine relationship to become more able to find and understand themselves. Such an approach implies a belief in people: what Maslow describes as 'a trust in the health-moving direction of most individuals'; a readiness to stand back, to respect and value people as they are and to help them to discover for themselves what they want to become.

Perhaps we are talking here about an ideal, about relationships and friendships which can help us all towards healthier and happier lives. In reality, how often do we encounter such ideal circumstances? How often, in particular, do people with learning difficulties find relationships which offer them trust, respect and acceptance? In this chapter we shall be looking at what is possible and trying to discover more about how the 'best' situations can come about.

Relationships and human development

There is no doubt that relationships *per se* are important for human development. For all of us, what we become as people, how we see ourselves and behave with others, is interwoven with the relationships we become involved in. If you are treated as a warm, interesting person to be with, then you are quite likely to see yourself in those terms and to behave accordingly. On the other hand, if people treat you as not particularly interesting or worthwhile, you will feel demoralised and probably show it in your behaviour. *It is difficult, if not impossible, to feel really good about yourself unless other people seem to feel good about you too.*

Without relationships we are more likely to experience stress and breakdown (Lynch, 1977), or to suffer from chronic physical ailments (Valliant, 1978). Good relationships help us to live longer, enjoy better physical and mental health, and feel happier (Argyle and Henderson, 1985). *In other words friends help us to stay healthy and happy.*

Close family ties seem to be the most important, but friends also help us to know ourselves. Particularly in adolescence, friendship is closely concerned with a developing self-awareness (Kon, 1981). In reviewing studies of adolescent friendship in several cultures, Kon considers a crucial question: Do the more intimate, personal, friendships of adolescence depend on the prior development of a clearer sense of personal identity and self-awareness? Or does that sense of self only emerge out of an experience of closer, more intimate relationships? He concludes that they should be seen, not as different stages of development, but as different aspects of the growth of an individual personality. *So the development of close relationships is part and parcel of our development as people.*

With support and affection from others we can come to believe in ourselves; with encouragement and help we can gain the confidence to try out and achieve new experiences and skills; with a network of friends we can find out more about how our environment works and can have more chance of exerting some control over it. Through personal relationships we can achieve more, know more, develop more, enjoy more, and become more fully a person.

Relationships and community living

The emphasis now is on living in the community, and this brings for many people with learning difficulties a new opportunity to develop relationships: ordinary relationships in ordinary settings. For others, and there are many, who have always lived in the community, it throws a new spotlight on existing relationships with families, friends and neighbours. The success or failure of personal relationships is perhaps the ultimate test of integration.

Nirje, one of the early exponents of a policy of normalisation, puts it like this:

'Isolation and segregation nourish public ignorance and prejudice, while integration and normalisation of the ways of life of smaller groups of mentally retarded people provide the opportunity for the ordinary human relationships which are the basis of understanding and social acceptance and integration of the individual.' Nirje, 1980, p.47.

The messages of normalisation demand for people with learning difficulties at least as good a chance in life as other people. They should not, by virtue of a disability, be deprived of ordinary possibilities for pleasurable life experiences, living circumstances and companions.

Making the structural and organisational changes and opening up some of the opportunities that go along with that process is an important step forward. But it is not the whole story. The truth is that living in the community is not a simple option. Families and individuals who have been doing it for countless years testify to the struggle against stereotyped attitudes and expectations, the exclusions and hurtfulness arising from ignorance and prejudice. Similarly those moving out of hospital as a part of the 'community-care' initiative frequently encounter attitudes of fear and rejection, often embedded in a 'not-in-our-street' type of reaction.

This is the other side of the story: the personal, experiential side of the structural and organisational changes we hear so much about. It is this personal side that will affect how each individual comes to understand him or herself, and will shape the experiences and opportunities that will help to form the individual personality. These are the relationship experiences that will critically affect

Maslow's 'process of growing into the best human being one can be'.

Where does the problem lie?

Researchers and clinicians have tended to focus on such relationships in ways which emphasise the problems for people with learning difficulties. For example, the process of developing personal relationships looked at under a microscope can be understood as a complex series of social and communication skills (e.g. Argyle, 1975). Such factors as the length, duration and timing of eye contact, the use of body language and body space, the timing and tone of contributions to a conversation, and the use of facial cues such as smiling, nodding, frowning etc. can all be seen to play a part in facilitating social interactions and enabling relationships to develop. Learning difficulties almost inevitably include difficulties, sometimes severe, with social and communication skills. Additional impairments of hearing, sight or physical development may further hamper the individual. When difficulties arise in relationships then, researchers and clinicians will see them as a direct result of poor social and communication skills – and the solution as primarily requiring a skills-training approach for the individual. The 'blame' for the relationship difficulties is seen as resting with the individual and any progress as dependent on his or her efforts to improve.

Another influential model for understanding relationships has been the 'social-exchange' theory (Homans, 1950; Thibaut and Kelley, 1959; Altman and Taylor, 1973). This model assumes that personal relationships will develop and be maintained when each partner feels they receive from the other an equal exchange of pleasure or resources. In other words the relationship is seen as mutually rewarding. This interpretation also seems to place the 'blame' for a failure to establish relationships on the individual who is seen as having less to offer. It seems to imply that if anyone is unfortunate enough to be for some reason on the sidelines, perhaps seen as somewhat different or as having less to offer in this 'market place' of social bartering, then it is essentially their problem.

The concept of normalisation has helped to shift our attention away from individual difficulties onto the creation of an adequate living environment with normal, valued life circumstances and opportunities for people. Unfortunately there is a tendency to misuse the concept to suggest that it is the individuals who must be 'normalised'. The strong traditions of clinical practice and the models of relationships outlined above encourage a return to pathological interpretations. We tend to see relationship problems as an individual disorder rather than as an outcome of a complex social process in which a particular group of people are being devalued and demoralised.

Limited opportunities?

By and large society has provided socially handicapping contexts for people with learning difficulties. That is to say, people who have more difficulty with learning than most of the population then find themselves facing a host of additional problems put in their way.

Intentions, of course, are largely philanthropic. The provision of alternative, segregated services and accommodation arose to protect vulnerable individuals from the demands of a society with which they seemed unable to cope. Such protective instincts, however, quickly lead to serious discrimination against individuals' rights to normal life experiences.

Not just segregated hospitals (Tizard, 1960 and 1964; Oswin, 1978; Ryan and Thomas, 1987) but also the separation from ordinary neighbourhood children involved in segregated schooling, the lack of work opportunities after school, the sheer impact of the label of 'mentally handicapped' on people's attitudes and behaviour towards them, have all contributed to limiting the chances of normal relationships and the normal social developments entailed.

Not only are relationships likely to be hampered by circumstances and the attitudes of others, but when good relationships occur, interpretations are likely to be stereotyped and prejudicial. A wish to get engaged or married will usually be seen as an immature, unrealistic passing fancy; the caring concern of one hospital resident for another may be seen as an attempt to dominate and take charge; friendships are likely to be interpreted as either superficial or one-sided; and natural parental concern will often be interpreted as over-protectiveness.

Positive relationships are thus demeaned by being frequently misrepresented or discounted; negative or difficult relationships on the other hand are seen inevitably as the fault of the individual with the disability. It is seldom considered that the individual may be lacking opportunities and appropriate support to develop personal relationships. It may be the social environment, rather than the individual, which is at fault (Brechin, 1981).

We offer restricted opportunities, we expect little, and we mis-interpret any relationships which do develop. Small wonder we have a situation which fosters one-sided relationships. We expect people with learning difficulties to be 'done unto' by others – at best to be protected, cared for, guided, supported, encouraged to learn and develop, tolerated and offered kindness. Atkinson and Ward (1986) outline a five-point guide to relationships. Their points include as one would expect: feeling safe with; feeling good with; learning from; benefiting from; but they also mention: giving to. They suggest that when relationships are all one-way, people can be described as having relationship 'vacancies'. Maybe we all like to feel we have something to give to others.

Some positive experiences

The truth is that two-way relationships have always been possible. Many parents over the years have testified to the sense of pleasure and fulfilment they have gained from their handicapped son or daughter (Collins and Collins, 1976; Hebden, 1985; Kaufman, 1976). To recognise this is not to deny the traumas, the sadness or the constant pressures, but simply to accept that there are rewards too. A mother in an Open University TV programme (Open University, 1986) says of her 18-year-old daughter who has Down's Syndrome: 'We truly were surprised by joy'. And later: 'She has taught us a new dimension of love because she loves so freely'. Even the mother described in the same Open University course, whose child was so severely handicapped she seemed unable to even recognise her parents, could still take pleasure from watching her daughter enjoy the wind in her hair or the sounds of music wafting over her (Atkinson and Ward, 1986).

Friendships outside the home, too, have always existed, with neighbourhood contacts, leisure activities, relatives and friends. Despite the lack of opportunities, the restrictions and stereotypes, good relationships have been possible (Atkinson and Ward, 1986; Edgerton, 1967, 1976b and 1984). With the increasing commitment to community living and to normalisation comes an obligation on us all to understand more about such relationships, how they operate, how they develop and how they can be encouraged and supported. People will only feel valued and fulfilled as individuals when they are valued through personal, reciprocal relationships. The challenge is to understand how to help that happen for everybody.

Case histories

Perhaps we can learn by looking at some examples, not exhaustively as a survey, but selectively, to find what people say about the quality and importance of relationships they have experienced.

Raun Kaufman was in most people's eyes a severely withdrawn autistic little boy. In his book, *To Love Is To Be Happy With* (Kaufman, 1976), his father describes the development of their relationship with their son as he and his wife confounded the specialists by helping him to progress beyond all expectations. Though somewhat over literary, the story is compelling and moving, as we follow the parents' struggle to discover and identify the crucial elements in their relationship with Raun.

First, their commitment and love were *unconditional*. They accepted what he could or could not offer them. If he was unable to respond to them, that was how he was. 'We wanted to help him reach the limit of his own possibilities, not impose on him standards from outside.' Their approach was *non-judgemental* and they were happy with him as their son. To make contact with Raun they had to come to know and understand him. Recognising his dignity as a person they sought to discover more about his way of operating. His mother spent hours each day with him participating in his experiences, become aware of the soothing, hypnotic effects gazing, spinning and rocking could have. 'We were beginning to come to grips with his world – without fear and anxiety but with love and acceptance and permissiveness.'

Slowly their commitment paid off, each step of the way being built on their intimate understanding of how he felt, how he experienced the world. Loving him meant leaving him alone in the true sense that Maslow implied – reaching through to him by helping him to become his own person.

Julie

John Swain's story of fostering Julie (Swain, 1977) has similiar themes.

'We became Julie's foster parents when she was 12 years old. At the time she weighed less than two stone. She was painfully thin, emaciated and without colour. She spat constantly, throwing out a ball of saliva every few seconds – within minutes a pool would be formed at her feet – as she walked she left a trail. In the same unconscious matter-of-fact way she masturbated. One hand was permanently fiddling between her legs, to the extent that she had worn holes through her clothing. She never ate spontaneously, would never eat sweets like other children, but reacted to food with little short of terror saying that she couldn't eat, that she was handicapped. In a similar way she was terrified of using the toilet, and could retain her faeces with a yogic control. Left to her own devices, Julie would stand with her head bent to the floor – recognising people by their shoes rather than their faces – and do little other than spit and masturbate.

'Julie had not developed the emotional self-sufficiency and independence required for healthy relationships with other people. She totally lacked self-esteem – seeing herself as an unlovable handicapped child with 'dirty habits'. She sought and expected rejection from other people, yet also used her behaviour problems to ensure her total dependence on others.

'She had lived in the care of a local authority from early childhood and had been passed from a nursery, to a children's home, to a hostel for mentally handicapped people, to a hospital for mentally handicapped people where we met her. In the hospital she was placed on what is called a "high dependency" ward where she lived with 25 profoundly and multiply handi-capped children, none of whom had any real speech, many being immobile, unable to feed themselves or use the toilet.

'Through our experiences with Julie, we have come to under-stand that being a foster parent to such a child requires far more than providing a family life – with all the important details that that entails – eating at the same table with family, using the same bath, the same toilet as the rest of the family. We found that there were a number of "simple" rules, at least they sounded simple but were very difficult to put into practice. We learnt them the hard way.

1. "Keep a balance between involvement and detachment."
   Julie needed love, not a patronising or sentimental attitude, but powerful emotions which demanded love in return. But we also needed detachment when we were rejected rather than loved in return.

2. "Where possible avoid a crisis."
   We found many ways of changing things (e.g. the position of the table at mealtimes or taking a day-trip to the seaside). It helped relieve the tension.

3. "Never to reject Julie."
   How do you show a child that though what she says or does is wrong, she herself is accepted and loved? Perhaps it is a matter of time more than anything else.

4. "Persevere."
   Keep going.

5. "Don't expect too much of Julie."
   We learnt to aim at and rejoice in small improvements, e.g. being able to drink from a cup without having to be persuaded to take each swallow.

6. "Keep a diary."

7. "Look for and accept regular relief."
   It was difficult to let others look after Julie, but we needed breaks.

Perhaps our last "rule" would be "don't believe in golden rules".
Brechin and Swain, 1987, pp. 8 and 9.

Again the themes emerge underlining what was needed to establish a relationship. *Time* and *commitment* were crucial. Julie's history of care was appalling, though not unusual, and trust could only be established over a long period of time. They too saw *unconditional acceptance* of Julie, herself, as crucial, as a starting point for trying to understand those elements of her behaviour which seemed to undermine her own chances of entering fully into a relationship of trust.

Common themes of time, commitment, participation and, above all, unconditional acceptance appear as the basic elements of coming to know and understand someone as a reciprocal relationship is established. These examples were parent/child relationships. What about close adult/adult relationships, particularly where sex or marriage is involved?

Meyers (1978) tells the story of his brother Roger's developing relationship and eventual marriage to Virginia Hensler. Through all the ups and downs it was interesting that the main stumbling blocks were not their own personal problems or relationship, about which they were quite relaxed, but the attitudes of other people. They did not have to receive sex education, or training in household skills, in order for them to develop a close personal relationship. Yet the need for this sort of preparation is often implied. Whelan and Speake (1979) for example seem to be suggesting in their book about adolescents that the development of particular interpersonal skills, including 'sexual knowledge and behaviour' is 'essential' before personal relationships can develop.

For Roger and Virginia, the relationship came first. They fell in love with each other. Then, of course, it made sense for them to think about how they could achieve their aim of getting married with all that this entailed. The pressures to fit in with society's view of normal married life are intense, and the sense of having to prove oneself at each hurdle in order to qualify for permission to marry can tend to become more important than the relationship itself.

Ann Craft's experience (e.g. Craft, 1986) suggests that often setting up home and marriage signifies a greater sense of independence and responsibility. In audio recordings made by her for the Open University course (Open University, 1986) David Sibbald talks about how his marriage helps him in feeling 'freer from my family, not so smothered, making our own decisions', and Sid Longmoor talking of his wife, Agnes, says: 'We have a life of our own – she used to be lonely in life, now I can have responsibility to give her love and affection'.

Finally in this section, it is important to recognise the increasing impact on relationships of the self-advocacy movement. Greater self-confidence and self-respect leads to an expectation of respect from the community at large.

'When I got involved in self-advocacy I began to recognise who I am, and how important I am to other people. And I never saw that before, up until now. Other people respect my opinion. A lot of things happened to me since I got involved. My whole personality changed around.' Bernard Carabello in Williams and Schoultz, 1982, p.78.

'I believe that our rights are very important, just as important as anybody else's rights. I believe we should be treated equal, have good jobs and let people *see* us.

'I believe it's happening. People are beginning to look at us and see us as people.' Larry Rice in Williams and Schoultz, 1982, p.75.

As more people have the courage to demand respect for themselves, others have to abandon entrenched, stereotyped responses. New styles of relationship are forged.

What are the risks?

One difficulty which can get in the way of the establishment of personal relationships is the fear of the risks involved. Relationships can be joyous and rewarding but they can also carry risks. Sometimes these risks loom so large in other people's minds that they seem to outweigh all the potential advantages. 'For their own good' people with learning difficulties may be protected from personal relationships with, inevitably, restrictive effects on their personal development.

A policy of normalisation carries with it greater risks. This does not have to imply a 'sink or swim' approach – all human beings need some protectors or allies (Edgerton, 1967, saw them as benefactors) who have a particular concern for their welfare – but nor can it avoid an implication of risk.

A sexual relationship can lead to pregnancy. It is difficult for some people to countenance either experience for people with learning difficulties. One mother in the Open University audio programme (*Ibid.*) described clearly how she felt she had to reach the stage first of genuinely accepting that her son had normal human rights – then his right to sexuality followed automatically. But what of pregnancy? Other people's rights, those of the unborn children, become involved.

The standard line tends to be that if counselling leads to 'informed consent' for sterilisation, then that is acceptable. If, however, informed consent is not really possible, then sterilisation is unacceptable. The catch-22 for the individual is that other preventive methods of birth control, whether the pill, personal restrictions or ultimately abortion, are likely to be used, which may in the end be more abusive of human choice and dignity and more distressing than sterilisation. Clearly this is an issue with a long debate to run. As with other human rights issues, it is not always clear which way to go when the rights of different individuals conflict.

Creating a relationship carries with it the risk of losing it. This may happen because friends 'fall out' or outgrow each other, because people move away, or through bereavement. Shirley Grant (not her real name) had a sadly typical experience (Atkinson and Ward, 1986). She lived alone with her mother, a fairly sheltered life, but within a well-established neighbourhood. When Mrs Grant developed cancer, nobody raised the subject of Shirley. Nor did anyone talk to Shirley about it. When her mother died it was a social worker who had only just met her who had to break the news, and arrange for her to move, away from home, to a hostel.

'Telling Shirley was awful. She was very upset. It seemed awful that she had suddenly lost everything – her Mum, her ATC friends, all the neighbours and friends she had known since childhood, the church she visited every week, and her home. Her whole life changed. I know I couldn't cope with all those losses at the same time – and I don't have the additional problems that Shirley has.'

In a misguided attempt to protect Shirley from distress, her sisters asked for her to be kept away from the hospital, away from the funeral and away from her home. She was thus denied the right to take part in the normal grieving and mourning process. People need time and support to come to terms with important losses in their lives. Denying or trying to hide away the fact of a death of a loved parent will not diminish the sense of loss, but may well make the process of recovery much slower and more difficult. Oswin (1981) has written about the experiences of bereavement of people with mental handicap. She found Shirley's situation to be all too common. People react like Shirley's sisters did because it is hard to cope with someone else's grief. Supporters need support too. And sometimes when understanding is limited, reactions may seem strange. Sadness and grief are not always shown in the same way. It may take all our powers of understanding to make sense of what someone else is experiencing.

A group of nursing staff recounted to me how a woman on their ward had shown no apparent grief when her father, a regular visitor, had died three months before. However much I questioned them, they remained convinced she felt no sense of sadness or loss. I met her that afternoon and her first words to me, a total stranger, were 'My daddy died'. After three months, whatever her lack of displayed emotion, the experience of that loss remained as the foremost experience in her mind, to be checked out and re-lived at every opportunity.

Recognising the pain involved in losing people whether through death, rejection or simply moving away, is the first step towards helping people to anticipate and cope with that loss. We all draw strength from others when they understand us and people with learning difficulties are no different. Such feelings of strength and support may come from close friends, from counsellors, or increasingly from self-help groups. CRUSE (The National Organisation for the Widowed and their Children) for example offers an opportunity for bereaved people to talk and share their feelings with people who will understand. Self-advocacy groups, too, may provide a setting in which people can work through their experiences of bereavement or their too-common experiences of rejection and prejudice, and gain confidence in their strength as individuals.

Developing relationships

Other relationships may be more casual, less intense, but none the less important. Leisure activities, work settings and casual neighbourhood interactions are often the 'stuff of life' and may be the area in which least protection can be afforded to people with learning difficulties. Exposure to possible ridicule, rejection or indifference is a painful possibility. Theoretical prediction and historical anecdote tend to be pessimistic about the possibilities, but more recent descriptive research studies have been able to show that positive relationships *can* be established.

Edgerton and Bercovici (1976) in their major follow-up study of people who had been living in the community over 10 years found that their major pre-occupations and satisfactions were with leisure-time activities, friends and families. Other, more conventional measures of success, were not felt to be important.

Atkinson (1986) describes the successful establishment of casual friendships and support networks and sees them as a way of interweaving formal and informal support in people's lives. Casual friendships require a context in which to occur. Anxieties and misconceptions need time to be overcome. 'We were very apprehensive at first – didn't know how to speak to her or what to talk about', says Renee in her account of getting to know Margaret at a keep fit class (Open University, 1986).

Regular contact, a context where there is a shared focus of interest and a framework to encourage a relationship through the early stages of anxiety on both sides seem to be the necessary preconditions for success. The use of leisure volunteers, link-up schemes and pathway schemes at work all offer ways forward (Gathercole, 1981; Jeffree and Cheseldine, 1984; McConkey and McCormack, 1983).

The situation or 'context' matters too. Argyle, Furnham and Graham (1981) devote a whole section of their book to considering how context changes can be used to facilitate the development of relationships. Environment itself is important in providing areas where a sense of home ground and privacy can develop, as well as places where group mixing occurs. Seating arrangements can be critical as studies in residential homes showed (Sommer and Ross, 1958; Ittleson, Proshansky and Rivlin, 1970). Very little social interaction occurs when seats are ranged along the walls of a room.

Who meets whom is important too. Argyle draws parallels with dating agencies, with single-parent organisations and with shared interest groups. 'People will like each other if they meet frequently, under rewarding circumstances, and are similar to one another in background, interests and values.' A focus on a shared activity or project is therefore a useful starting point. McConkey, putting some of the theories into practice (1983), found friendships could develop through shared involvement where people came together as equals to work on community projects. Cook (1977) suggested that, particularly where people are socially unskilled for whatever reason, 'the more joint displacement activities organised for them, the better the chances of friendship formation'. In other words, focus attention on something else and let the relationship take care of itself.

On types of activities, many suggestions emerge. Argyle mentions hobbies, and political or religious activities; the Conference on Informal Supports (1985) mentioned as examples gardening, weightlifting, home maintenance and fishing; Peter, on one of the Open University course audio-tapes (Open University, 1986), mentions building his friendship with Mike through activities including going for a drink, visiting a nearby town, a motor show, a football match, an outing for a birthday meal, bowling, an exhibition, a Christmas shopping trip to *Asda* and a simple walk to the park.

The activities exist, the know-how exists, but does the commitment of ordinary people exist? It was argued earlier that up to a point it always has existed. With more community-based living for more individuals with learning difficulties, the question is simply: Will the commitment spread to become a natural way for society to operate? Maslow (1973) is optimistic about what can be achieved:

'On the whole I think it is fair to say that human history is a record of the ways in which human nature has been sold short. The highest possibilities of human nature have practically always been underrated.'

The creation of a society in which people value each other for what they are, without seeking first and foremost 'to interfere, to control, to change, to improve', would bring rewards for us all. Not only those with learning difficulties would gain from a greater sense of humanity. Rather than arguing about whether or not 'ideals' can ever be achieved, we can use what we know already to create a climate where positive personal relationships flourish, and where individuals achieve a sense of personal fulfilment.

Further reading

1. Altman, I., Taylor, D. A., *Social Penetration: The Development of*

Interpersonal Relationships (NY, Holt, Rinehart and Winston, 1973).
2. Argyle, M., *Bodily Communication* (London, Methuen, 1975).
3. Argyle, M., Furnham, A., Graham, J. A., *Social Situations* (Cambridge University Press, 1981).
4. Argyle, M., Henderson, M., *The Anatomy of Relationships* (Penguin Books, 1985).
5. Atkinson, D., 'Engaging Competent Others: A study of the support networks of people with mental handicap', *British Journal of Social Work*, vol. 16, 1986 supplement pp.83–101.
6. Atkinson, D., Ward, L., *Living and Learning*, Book 1 in *Mental Handicap: Patterns for Living*. An open learning pack for parents and care staff. (Open University Press, 1986).
7. Atkinson, D., Ward, L., *A Part of the Community: Social Integration and Neighbourhood Networks* (London, CMH, 1986).
8. Brechin, A., 'Behaviourism and the Environment', in Brechin, A., Liddiard, P., Swain, J., (eds.) *Handicap in a Social World* (Hodder and Stoughton, 1981).
9. Brechin, A., Swain, J., *Changing Relationships: Shared Action Planning with People with Mental Handicap* (From Open University (1986) op. cit., Harper and Row, 1987).
10. Conference on Informal Supports, 1985, *Personal Relationships for Persons with Developmental Disabilities* (De-Institutionalisation Task Force, Residential Inc.).
11. Collins, M., Collins, D., *Kith and Kids* (Souvenir Press, 1976).
12. Cook, M., 'The Social Skill Model and Interpersonal Attraction', in Duck, S., (ed.) *Theory and Practice in Interpersonal Attraction* (NY and London, Academic Press, 1977).
13. Craft, A., *Mental Handicap and Sexuality: Issues and Perspectives* (Tunbridge Wells, Costello Press, 1986).
14. Duck, S., Gilmour, R., (eds.) *Developing Personal Relationships* (London, Academic Press, 1981).
15. Edgerton, R. B., *The Cloak of Competence* (Berkeley: University of California Press, 1967).
16. Edgerton, R. B., Bercovici, S. M., 'The Cloak of Competence: years later', *American Journal of Mental Deficiency*, vol. 80, (1976) No. 5, pp.485–97.
17. Edgerton, R. B., Bollinger, M., Herr, B., 'The Cloak of Competence: After two decades', *American Journal of Mental Deficiency*, vol. 88 (1984) No. 4, pp.345–51.
18. Gathercole, C., *Residential Alternatives for Adults who Are Mentally Handicapped, vol. 4: Leisure, Social Integration and Volunteers* (Kidderminster, BIMH, 1981).
19. Hebden, J., *She'll Never Do Anything, Dear* (London, Souvenir Press, 1985).
20. Homans, G. C., *The Human Group* (London, Routledge and Kegan Paul, 1950).

21. Ittleson, W. H., Proshansky, H. M., Rivlin, L. G., 'The Environmental Psychology of the Psychiatric Ward', in Proshansky *et al.* (eds.) *Environmental Psychology* (NY, Holt, Rinehart and Winston, 1970).
22. Jeffree, D., Cheseldine, S., *Let's Join In* (Souvenir Press, 1984).
23. Kaufman, B. N., *To Love Is To Be Happy With* (Human Horizons series, Souvenir Press (E and A) Ltd., 1976).
24. Kon, I. A., 'Adolescent Friendship' in Duck, S., Gilmour, R., (ed.) *Developing Personal Relationships* (Academic Press: London, 1981).
25. Lynch, J. J., *The Broken Heart: The Medical Consequences of Loneliness* (New York, Basic Books, 1977).
26. Maslow, A. H., *The Further Reaches of Human Nature* (Pelican Books, 1973).
27. McConkey, R., McCormack, B., *Breaking Barriers: Educating People about Disability* (Souvenir Press, 1983).
28. Meyers, R., *Like Normal People* (Souvenir Press, 1978).
29. Nirje, B., 'The Normalisation Principle', in Flynn, J., Nitsch, K., (eds.) *Normalisation, Social Integration and Community Services* (University Park Press, 1980).
30. Open University, *Mental Handicap: Patterns for Living*. An open learning pack for parents and care staff. (Learning Materials Service Office, Centre for Continuing Education, The Open University, Walton Hall, Milton Keynes, MK7 6AA. (Open University Press, 1986).
31. Oswin, M., *Children Living in Long-Stay Hospitals* (London, Spastics International Medical Publications, Heinemann Medical Books, 1978).
32. Oswin, M., *Bereavement and Mentally Handicapped People* (London, Kings' Fund Centre, 1981).
33. Rogers, C., *On Becoming a Person* (London, Constable, 1961).
34. Rogers, C., *Client Centred Therapy* (Boston: Houghton Mifflin, 1951).
35. Ryan, J., Thomas, F., *The Politics of Mental Handicap* (Penguin Books, 1980).
36. Sommer, R., Ross, H., 'Social Interaction on a Geriatric Ward', *International Journal of Social Psychiatry*, vol. 4 (1958), pp.128–33.
37. Swain, J., *Spit Once for Luck: Fostering Julie, a Disturbed Child* (Elek, 1977)
38. Thibaut, J. W., Kelley, H. H., *The Sociology of Groups* (NY, John Wiley and Sons, 1959).
39. Tizard, 'Residential Care of Mentally Handicapped Children', *BMJ*, vol. I (1960), pp.1,041–6.
40. Tizard, *Community Services for the Mentally Handicapped* (Oxford University Press, 1964).
41. Valliant, G. E., 'Natural History of Male Psychological

Health: VI Correlates of successful marriage and fatherhood', *American Journal of Psychiatry*, vol 135 (1978), pp.653–59.

42. Whelan, E., and Speake, B., *Learning to Cope*, (Souvenir Press, London, 1979).

43. Williams, P., Shoultz, B., *We Can Speak for Ourselves* (Human Horizons, Souvenir Press, 1982).

PART THREE

Community care and some special groups

CHAPTER 11

Profound retardation and multiple handicap: a life in the community

Loretto Lambe
Co-ordinator MENCAP PRMH Project

For community care to become a reality for one special group of people, those with profound retardation and multiple handicaps, there has to be in existence a full local support network to help families maintain their son or daughter in the home or in locally-based residential care. This support by definition must be multi-disciplinary and geared to respond to the parent's and carer's needs.

Who are people with profound and multiple handicaps? Where are they? What are their needs and those of their carers? A recent national postal survey undertaken by MENCAP's Profound Retardation and Multiple Handicap (PRMH) Project throws some light on these questions. Before reviewing some of the main findings from the survey report, Hogg, Lambe *et al.* (1987), it would be helpful to clarify the definition of profound retardation and multiple handicap.

Definition

While categories for people have become unfashionable during the past few years, it is still necessary to identify people with particular patterns of handicap if we are to provide specialised services for such groups. There is no generally agreed characterisation of people who are profoundly retarded and multiply impaired (Fryers, 1984). For the purpose of this chapter the definition used is that adopted by the MENCAP PRMH Project. This is broadly in line with international systems of classification in the field of retardation. With respect to children, an Intelligence Quotient below 20 (IQ<20) was adopted. This implies that the Mental Age (MA) of the child is approximately one-fifth or less of his or her Chronological Age (CA), e.g. a 15-year-old with a MA of three years or less. In addition, one or more impairments to hearing, vision or physical functioning which significantly reduces adaptive behaviour must be present. With respect to young people and adults over 15 years of age, the same general definition has been adopted, i.e.,

IQ<20 and one or more sensory and/or physical impairments. However, here it is assumed that beyond a chronological age of 15 years, increase in an individual's MA will be modest and, therefore, a fixed MA<3 years is specified.

As with any definition of this population, problems can be identified in the criteria chosen. Assessment of IQ and MA in profoundly impaired people is extremely difficult. In addition, we do not specify exactly what is meant by ' . . . a significant reduction in adaptive behaviour'. Ideally a definition based on marked reductions in adaptive behaviour, i.e., a functional definition, would be adopted. However, as Fryers (1984) points out, no generally agreed definition yet exists, and like him, the Project adopted the more widely used categories reflecting general developmental level.

One strength of the definition, however, is that it embraces the most handicapped individuals who make up the majority of the 'special needs' population in schools, Adult Training Centres/ Special Education Centres (ATCs/SECs) and hospitals, as well as some more able people who may adapt to settings demanding higher abilities. Initial work by the MENCAP PRMH Project indicated that the definition adequately communicates to most care givers the Project's target population, i.e., parents and care givers of children and adults with profound retardation and multiple handicaps.

Size of population

An exact estimate of the prevalence of people with profound retardation and multiple impairments is difficult to establish. The few studies reviewed by Fryers (1984) on prevalence of profound retardation (as defined above) suggest 1/1,000 of the school-age population. Jacobson, Sutton and Janicki (1985) show that there is a higher rate of mortality for adults who are profoundly retarded than for more able retarded people and that prevalence will therefore decrease with age relative both to more able people with mental handicap and to the general population. In other words, mortality will remain higher for people with profound retardation throughout the age span and there will be proportionally fewer such individuals at each age level.

Not all people with profound retardation will have additional impairments, but there is little doubt that an IQ<20 is associated with high probability of physical or sensory handicaps. Dupont (1981), for example, reports that over 80 per cent of people with profound retardation do have at least one such serious impairment. Overall, then, we can anticipate that the number of people in the population within this definition would reflect prevalence well below 1/1,000, i.e., substantially below the figure of 49,155 such an estimate would yield on the basis of the 1981 population figure of 49,154, 687 for England and Wales (OPCS 1984). Indeed, a figure of two-thirds of this number would seem more realistic, i.e., 32,000. This accords with the sum of estimates for schools, ATCs/SECs, hospitals that can be made: i.e., 8,000 (Hogg and Sebba 1986), 3,000 (Whelan and Speake 1985) and 13,000 respectively (hospital population based on assumption of just under one-third of this population of 40,000 being PRMH). This total of 24,000 allows a margin of 8,000 for people who are PRMH but who may be living in the community at home or in hostels and not at present attending schools or ATCs/SECs. It must be emphasised that this figure is at best an informed guess and was employed to guide the sampling in the survey.

As children, such people will generally be found in schools for children with severe learning difficulties, while many young people and adults in their middle years are attending ATCs/SECs. Those in school and ATCs/SECs will be living at home or in statutory or voluntary residential hostels or group homes. Many adults will also be in long-stay hospitals, particularly the ageing (55–64 years) and elderly (> 65 years).

The MENCAP Survey

Aims

The objectives of the MENCAP survey were threefold. First, to identify families and other care givers whose sons, daughters or charges were profoundly retarded and multiply handicapped. Second, to establish the needs of these people through direct questions about their lives and the activity of caring for a person with such severe impairments to development and function. Third, to propose ways in which MENCAP might meet some of these needs, and to provide information for those working in the wider field of mental handicap services which would give them guidance as to what improvements in services might be effected.

In line with the objective of this volume we will focus here on the responses of parents and foster parents who had living with them at home the child or adult with profound retardation and multiple handicaps on whom they completed the questionnaire. Approximately 350 questionnaires reporting on children provide the basis for this analysis, and 175 returns on adults.

Characteristics of survey population

The majority of people who were the subjects of questionnaires were so delayed in development and lacking in functional self-help skills that they fell within the definition of profound retardation. The majority, too, had additional physical and sensory handicaps as required by the definition. Inspection of almost any of the figures presented in Hogg, Lambe *et al*. (1987) will show that with respect to abilities, performance falls with great consistency at the lower end of all scales. As well as developmental status and additional impairments, many in both child and adult samples had further medical problems, including epilepsy, as well as behaviour problems.

Caring at home: educational and social provision

In this section a number of issues related to caring at home will be covered. These will include education and therapeutic needs, behaviour problems and use of leisure-time. Interactions between the various problem areas can create an overwhelming complex of pressures. Here we identify some of the elements that need to be dealt with on the assumption that if they are alleviated, benefits will accrue which range far beyond the immediate specific intervention.

EDUCATIONAL AND THERAPEUTIC NEEDS

At the most fundamental level, parents have expressed the need for direct assistance with respect to the nature of the intellectual and physical handicaps displayed by their sons and daughters. Of primary concern is the wish to enhance that most fundamental of human capacities: language. In both child and adult samples a majority of sons and daughters were reported as making no more than babbling sounds, while a substantial number of parents believed that their offspring did not communicate at all. For 78 per cent of children's parents and 61 per cent of the adults', the main area of educational activity in which advice would be found helpful was language and communication. Clearly such information could come through school-based workshops or advice sessions from teaching staff or through a direct input to the home. In both settings, a speech therapist could provide such advice. It is clear, however, that many parents do not see the speech therapist as the most likely source of this help. Against the figures of 78 and 61 per cent noted above, only 46 per cent of children's parents and 38 per cent of adults' indicated that advice from a speech therapist would be helpful and only around a quarter that practical assistance was required. Of these, some would doubtless be looking to the speech therapist not for assistance with respect to language and communication, but for help with feeding and other oral activities. Indeed, 53 per cent of children's parents and 31 per cent of parents of adults indicated that advice on feeding would be welcome: an unsurprising figure given the low level of self-feeding ability reported.

Taken together, these statistics show a clear demand for advice and assistance in developing 'oral skills' related to feeding and to language, though non-oral communication such as signing must also be included in this requirement. While parents look to the speech therapist for advice and help, it is clear their expectations extend beyond this profession to those providing educational and training services.

During the summer of 1987, the MENCAP PRMH Project ran a workshop in Manchester, 'Communication and Feeding for Parents and Carers'. Throughout the course of the workshop, the handicapped person, as well as any siblings, were cared for in a special leisure scheme, described below. Thus the parents/carers were free to attend the workshop in the knowledge that their son or daughter was being cared for in a stimulating environment. The workshop, the first of series, was run as a pilot in Manchester and its effectiveness is at present being evaluated. It is anticipated that the model developed will be used by MENCAP and others to run similar workshops throughout the country.

As well as low levels of communicative development, we also find gross motor skill restricted, for most respondents' sons and daughters, to the very early developmental milestones. This reflects in large measure the high prevalence of the major additional impairment reported, i.e., physical impairment. Considerably more parents of children than of adults had been offered advice from a physiotherapist; 75 per cent compared with 39 per cent. A similar discrepancy was also noted for receipt of practical assistance: 22 per cent and 3 per cent respectively. The excessively low input for adults cannot be accounted for by a relatively lower prevalence of physical impairments in this group and must be seen as a failure of service delivery. Certainly the need for advice and demonstration from a physiotherapist was reported by 37 per cent of parents of children and 20 per cent of parents of adults, while practical help would have been welcomed by 29 per cent and 16 per cent, respectively. Already a majority of parents of children are spending more than one hour a day on exercise and stimulation, as is a substantial minority of adults' parents. Where, as in the majority of families, advice is not being received, the quality of these activities could undoubtedly be enhanced. In addition, basic information on handling and positioning could be critical in avoiding deformities in individuals with handicaps and in avoiding injury and fatigue in their parents.

Distinctions between gross and fine motor development, i.e, use of hands, is somewhat artificial, as it is widely agreed that the development of adaptive motor competence involves the complementary development of postural control *and* eye-hand co-ordination. Thus, the physiotherapist may well be involved in working in this total motor development area as well as being concerned with gross activities related to bodily movement. Similarly, teachers and ATC/SEC staff will have an important role to play in this area. However, the occupational therapist will be particularly concerned with finer motor activities which embrace educational, self-help and leisure activities. Help with teaching use of hands was the second greatest need expressed by children's parents (59 per cent) and the fourth greatest noted by adults' parents (42 per cent), suggesting an important role for the occupational therapist. Parents had received less advice, but more practical assistance, from occupational than from speech therapists. Their expressed need for advice was slightly less for speech therapy input, with just under a third of each sample requesting this. However, the need for practical assistance was about the same for both samples with respect to occupational and speech therapy help: in the region of a quarter of each sample. As noted above, interventions related to hand use would have implications for some of the other self-help areas of concern to parents, e.g. washing, care of clothing etc.

The preceding paragraphs clearly show the need for an increase in such home intervention and point to the professions who might be involved. For language and communication, gross motor development, and for hand use, teachers and ATC/SEC staff will play a central role in co-ordinating their own activities with those of family members. Specialised input for each area will also come from speech, occupational and physiotherapists.

Wider issues of service provision also present themselves when we consider the role of schools and ATCs/SECs in providing such services. It is clear that the transition from school to ATC/SEC, when such an option is available, can be a matter of concern for a number of parents. The fear exists that a poorer service is provided in the training establishment than was offered at school and that gains made will subsequently be lost. The onus clearly rests with centre staff and local authorities to develop demonstrably adequate provision for people with profound retardation and multiple handicaps in order to alleviate these concerns.

DEALING WITH BEHAVIOUR PROBLEMS

For both child and adult samples in the survey a remarkably consistent picture regarding behaviour problems emerged with respect to both the prevalence and nature of the difficulties. In the region of three quarters of all families report one or more behaviours they regard as a problem, with the parents of adults indicating in general greater difficulties. For a majority of those who do report behaviour problems more than one such behaviour is noted. As would be anticipated from the literature on this topic the most likely behaviours to be exhibited relate to repetitive or stereotyped behaviour and/or making disruptive sounds or noises. When asked directly in which areas assistance is required, help in dealing with behaviour problems is the second choice (after communication) for adults' parents (56 per cent) and fifth choice (equal with leisure) for children's parents (49 per cent). This difference between the samples is consistent with the reported greater prevalence of behaviour problems among adults than among children. So pervasive can such behaviour problems be, that activities in a variety of areas of life can be affected. In addition, the more broadly based educational and therapeutic activities described in the preceding section will also be precluded or undermined. This, as with any such educational and therapeutic activities, must be regarded as a major concern for those trying to assist the families.

The MENCAP PRMH Project will also run workshops on behaviour problems. Professor Chris Kiernan, who has worked in this area for a number of years, and is involved in developing techniques and strategies for dealing with problem behaviours, will be directing the first such workshop. Again, it is anticipated that the model adopted and materials developed will be made available to others to mount similar exercises.

LEISURE ACTIVITIES

Hogg, Lambe *et al.* (1987) noted that ' . . . parents in both groups see leisure as part of their sons' and daughters' lives that merits an investment of time'. They also noted the emphasis on what might be regarded as passive pursuits such as watching television or listening to music, though cautioning against assuming that this is necessarily very different from the way the rest of the population passes its time. However, they pointed out that most parents do attempt to produce a balanced diet by complementing passive activities with more active ones such as toy or social play.

The willingness to commit time to organising leisure and the thought given to the form it takes is reflected in the importance leisure assumes when parents were asked directly in which areas help would be welcome. For parents of adults, leisure was third choice (50 per cent) after communication and behaviour problems. A similar proportion of children's parents (49 per cent) placed leisure in fifth place (equal with the need for help with behaviour problems). When asked about social provision, advice on leisure activities also emerged as a consistent strain of concern. While never figuring as the major priority in this area (a position occupied by advice on future residential placement, benefits and family or emotional problems) it emerged as the major second and third choice priorities in both groups.

It can be inferred, then, that while leisure activity does not figure as a major preoccupation in the way that communication or future residential placements do, it is a very important concern of parents and one which must be dealt with in any comprehensive system of support and provision. To this should be added the point that for people with mental handicap, as with the rest of the population, the majority of their time is not spent in formal education, training or employment. Most of it is free time. In addition, if parents were helped to use this time in an enjoyable and beneficial way, there would be less pressure on schools to divert resources during the school day to activities that reduce the already limited time available for implementing the basic curriculum.

There are already a number of leisure initiatives for people with mental handicap. Not all of these cater for people with profound and multiple handicaps. However, some of the voluntary and statutory agencies are now looking at the needs of this group. The Save the Children Fund's *Playtrac Project*, initially set up to develop play for multiply handicapped people in long-stay hospitals, has now widened its brief and is developing play activities for people living in the community. The National Federation of Gateway Clubs (leisure clubs for people with mental handicap) and the MENCAP PRMH Project have set up a joint working party with a brief to develop leisure initiatives for people with multiple impairments and to produce a training pack for use by volunteers and parents. Again, this will be piloted in the North West, evaluated, and then disseminated throughout the Gateway and MENCAP network.

Since 1985 the PRMH Project has developed hydrotherapy/leisure schemes in Manchester. These were run as pilots in the first year but are now funded by the Recreational Services Department as part of their normal services. Similar schemes based on this model have now been set up in other areas. The PRMH Project has also developed special leisure schemes for multiply handicapped children. These are run during the school summer holiday periods, a time at which parents reported greatest difficulty in coping. All of the schemes described above have two common aims: first, to involve the handicapped person in leisure activities suitable to their very special needs; second, and equally as important, to offer respite to families and carers.

Caring at home: medical and paramedical support

To sustain a person with multiple handicaps in the community, it is essential that they and their families have access to good medical and paramedical services. Medical information to families in general cannot be regarded as adequate. In the MENCAP survey, of the 52 per cent of parents of children who had received sufficient medical information, 26 per cent considered it unintelligible. Comparable figures for the adult sample are 32 and 65 per cent. Thus, in a majority of instances in both samples, parents had not received sufficient *and* intelligible information, a situation that was appreciably worse in the case of the adult sample. While there has been improvement over the years in the adequacy of medical information given to parents of children who are multiply handicapped, there is clearly a long way to go in developing communication between parents and medical practitioners in this area. To this point might be added the fact that where positive judgements were given, written comments often qualified these by indicating that the judgement related to a specific, individual GP or paediatrician, rather than to the profession as a whole.

General Practitioners or consultants are not the only medical staff from whom families require help. Advice on nursing care in the home was requested by 14 and 16 per cent of children's and adults' parents respectively, with eight per cent in each sample indicating that practical help on a regular basis was needed. Though these figures are relatively small when compared with some other needs expressed, they are of some significance given the medical complications that can co-exist with the various handicapping conditions.

The degree of visual handicap, if any, of the respondents' sons and daughters was not known in, respectively, eight and seven per cent of cases, while their hearing status was not known in three and five per cent of cases. When information is available, however, it is frequently inadequate, as is shown by the fact that 27 per cent of children's parents and 14 per cent of those of adults indicated they required advice from a specialist on vision, and 17 and six per cent did so with regard to hearing.

It seems axiomatic that reliable and up-to-date information on the sensory abilities of people with profound retardation and multiple handicaps is critical to all educational activities we might wish to undertake. This is the case whether we consider language development with its dependence on hearing, or manipulative activities in which eye-hand co-ordination is central. Even in less obvious areas such as leisure this information is crucial if we are to select in an appropriate way. While techniques of assessment which can be used by teachers, trainers and other non-specialists do exist and should be employed (see Sebba, 1987), regular specialist assessments should be available to the families as a matter of course.

Similarly, where dietary difficulties exist or are suspected, specialist advice will also be required, as indicated by 11 per cent of children's parents and eight per cent of adults'. Of special interest with regard to medically-related advice was the finding that 40 per cent of both samples required dental advice. Again, the MENCAP PRMH Project is planning workshops for parents and carers on this important topic.

The above clearly shows that people with multiple handicaps, their families and carers, require help and advice from the medical and paramedical professionals throughout their lives. This support, in the main, is not at present forthcoming for a number of families. While it is desirable that people with mental handicap should wherever possible use generic services, access to specialist services may have to be facilitated by families' social workers and key workers to ensure that those who need them are made aware of these services.

Caring at home: support and provision

The background of general educational, therapeutic and medical information that parents require, discussed above, relates in a direct way to the particular pattern of impairments displayed by people with profound retardation and multiple handicaps. Of equal importance is a range of social and environmental provision which is critical to the life of the family.

Services that offer families support in the home are crucial in helping them maintain their handicapped son or daughter in the community. The Birmingham Multi-Handicap Group offers such a service to families (McCorry, 1987). This Group, a voluntary organisation, has set up a service that offers preventative support to families. They match the family with trained carers, who go into the home at short notice any time of the day or night, to take over the care. A minimum of 2 hours relief can be promised to each family each month, with unlimited extra emergency provision, if required. This home-based intervention allows families regular respite and reduces the need for long-term residential provision. The expansion in this service reflects the satisfaction of families who have been involved.

NIMROD, a comprehensive service for people with mental handicap and their families in west Cardiff, offers services in addition to, rather than instead of, existing services. The central component of the service is the Individual Planning (IP) System (Humphreys, Lowe and de Paiva, 1986). Each client is allocated a Keyworker, who prepares for and co-ordinates the IP meeting. At each IP meeting, decisions regarding the handicapped person's present and future needs are made. These include the setting of skill goals for the client and for service personnel. Although the NIMROD service deals with some clients with severe mental and physical handicaps, the majority are less disabled. However, the keyworker system developed by NIMROD could be adopted by other service providers helping families caring for a profoundly multiply handicapped person.

SHORT AND LONG-TERM RESIDENTIAL PROVISION

Hogg, Lambe *et al.* (1987) noted that the level of contact with social workers was high in both groups, with the main need being advice and assistance in gaining short or long-term residential placement (56 and 76 per cent of the child and adult sample parents respectively). While satisfaction with the advice was high in both groups (child sample 72 per cent and adult sample 76 per cent), advice on future residential placement remained the major area of social provision in which parents required further guidance, particularly, as we might expect, for the parents of adults. Adults' parents fared somewhat better than children's with respect to short-term residential care, though only about half the parents in each group deemed such provision was readily available and only just over half in each sample were *satisfied* with the quality of the care. In both samples a majority of parents who were planning future long-term residential accommodation had not yet found a placement. Parents in both groups, but particularly the parents of children, favoured normalised, community-based accommodation.

There is a clear need for parents to receive advice and guidance on residential placement. Professionals in a position to provide such advice need to have adequate information on available provision. Of equal importance, however, is the availability of high quality, community-based residential provision geared to the particular needs of people with profound retardation and multiple impairments.

There are however, models of good practice which should be noted here. The Barnardo's Croxteth Park Project in Liverpool offers an Intensive Support Unit and demonstrates that profoundly mentally handicapped children can be cared for by residential social workers in ordinary houses using facilities and services already available in the community (Alaszewski, Ong and Lovett, 1986). The project cares for eight children in four houses in a desirable area of Liverpool. All of the children previously lived in hospitals.

MENCAP's Homes Foundation, a scheme that provides small group homes in the 'community for people with mental handicap has recently widened its brief to consider the needs of people with multiple handicaps. Until now Homes Foundation has not catered for this group of people, but discussions are currently taking place to develop and plan some pilot schemes for people with multiple handicaps. With respect to more able people with profound retardation, Saxby and Felce (1986) have evaluated the success of transition from hospital to ordinary dwellings in Andover and have explored a model of provision and staff training aimed at maintaining a high quality service. Clear improvements in functional behaviour were found, with residents taking part more appropriately in a variety of activities. Saxby and Felce clearly show that such improvement is not simply a function of a person's intelligence, but that the organisation of the homes, their design and material environment, and the performance of staff, all have important influences.

As well as long-term residential schemes, a number of pioneering fostering schemes for people with profound retardation and multiple handicaps have been developed over the past few years. Barnardo's Professional Foster Care Service is one such scheme (Wolfarth, Dodson, Dixon, Kendall, Hardy, 1985): 'The aim of the scheme is to recruit, train and support foster-parents for children who by reason of mental, physical or emotional handicap, or a combination of these, it has proved very difficult or impossible to find regular foster-parents for in the past. The professional element in the description of the foster-parents indicates a higher expectation on the agency's part of the foster-parent through involvement in training programmes, implementation of programmes, and in their relationship to the agency.' (p.11.) Comparable schemes have been developed elsewhere in the country, for example, the Family Fostering Scheme set up by Manchester Social Services.

While models of such good practice do exist throughout the country and publicity of such ventures is of value in guiding local authorities who are failing to make such provision, there is a long way to go before such provision becomes the norm.

Advice on benefits and financial requirements

Hogg, Lambe *et al.* (1987) describe the financial benefits being received by parents. In the region of three quarters of both samples received day and night attendance allowance and mobility allowance. Of those not receiving full attendance allowance, most of the remainder received day time allowance. It was evident, however, that a wide range of additional costs were incurred and that income and benefits were insufficient to meet needs without severe financial pressures. Seventy-nine per cent of children's parents and 69 per cent of adults' noted that additional financial help towards heating costs was needed, while 64 and 65 per cent respectively needed help with laundry costs. Assistance with the cost of special equipment, transport and help in the home were also required by substantial percentages of parents in both groups.

Forty-two per cent of the parents of children and 35 per cent of those of adults had received advice or benefits from social workers. Of those who received such information, 63 per cent in the former sample expressed satisfaction, as did 83 per cent in the latter. In response to direct questions on the needs for such advice, however, guidance on benefits still emerged as a major requirement. It seems that much remains to be done in an area in which it should be possible to ensure that *all* families have at their disposal information which will permit them to claim *all* their entitlements.

The financial implications of having a son or daughter with profound retardation and multiple handicaps needs to be considered from two standpoints. First, it is essential that appropriate advice is given on available benefits in order that support from such sources of income is optimised. Second, consideration must be given to meeting those essential needs that have financial consequences, such as adequate heating, which enable the parents to maintain their son or daughter in their home. A more detailed study would be welcome in which a full evaluation of the costs of such maintenance could be made and compared with the actual cost of statutory provision in a community-based residential establishment.

To this consideration must be added a comment on the making of financial provision for the future of a son or daughter with handicaps. Information on the setting up of trusts and making of wills is of some importance. Sixty per cent of children's parents and 54 per cent of those of adults indicated that information would be welcome. Confirmation of this need was recently given when over 350 people came to a meeting organised by the PRMH Project to discuss these issues.

Housing requirements

The issue of providing suitable and adequate housing for families caring for a person with profound retardation and multiple handicaps is not unrelated to the previous section, in that modification to a house or flat will usually have finanical implications. The inadequacy of their accommodation for many families is shown by the fact that in the MENCAP survey 63 per cent of children's parents and 55 per cent of adults' had moved house, received a grant for modifying the house, or *both*, at some time in the past. In reality these figures are underestimates since a number of families indicated they had made modifications at their own expense. Despite the large number who have made such changes, many problems remained with respect to access and movement within the house (e.g. narrow hall and stairs). From the point of view of the families almost 20 per cent in both samples see the solution to existing problems as a move to another house. Many, however, indicated very specific modifications such as, for example, installation of a stair lift (23 per cent of children's parents and 12 per cent of adults').

The impression gained, therefore, is that it is not advice *per se* that is required but financial assistance in making specific alterations to the home.

Travel and mobility

Both local and wider travel consistently present problems for families in both samples. For local travel, a majority in both samples use a wheelchair either all or part of the time. For a very substantial majority, public transport is not an option and a private car or taxi is the preferred mode of travel.

The factors that will lead to improvements in family mobility obviously tend to be very specific with regard to the situations that result in difficulties. For example, 43 per cent of children's parents and 52 per cent of adults' require improvement to the wheelchair to enhance mobility, while better access to local shops and services would further improve the situation. For around half of both samples, ownership of a private car would be helpful, while for about a quarter modification of the existing car would be advantageous. With respect to public transport, availability of assistance and modifications to seating are also noted as desirable. For these improvements to be effected, it is clear that there must be strategic changes in the whole approach to access and mobility involving local authorities, shop-keepers, cinema chains and theatres, and bus, train and airline companies.

Improved mobility can result, too, from the changing competence of the people with handicaps. Obviously improvements in the ability to walk will enhance the situation as will the elimination of behaviour problems, an important factor in making travel difficult for nearly 40 per cent of both samples.

The family and the community

Given the plethora of problems and needs described above, and the more general psychological consequences of having a child with handicaps in the family, it is inevitable that stresses can be placed on families with which they have difficulty in coping. Over half of each sample (55 per cent children's parents and 57 per cent of adults') had had contact with a social worker in order to deal with family stress or problems. Of these, 69 per cent in both groups had found such contact helpful. Advice on family or emotional problems was a major concern of parents in both samples, after the more practical issues of advice on residential placement and benefits.

In the present context of services it is likely to be the social worker who is primarily going to assist in family problems, though in some situations referral to clinical psychologists or psychiatrists may ensue. Members of voluntary agencies, including self-help groups with their unique insight into common problems, also have a crucial role to play.

Hogg, Lambe *et al.* (1987) concentrated on parents but did ask some questions about the impact on brothers and sisters of having a family member with such serious handicaps. While noting that parents' reports on their children's feelings might not be as valid as a direct sounding of the children themselves, it nevertheless seemed important to collect such information. It emerged that while school life was little affected, friendships were more adversely influenced and parents do report considerable disturbance in the siblings in the child sample. Advice on how to cope was required for 18 per cent of siblings in the children's sample and 11 per cent in the adult sample, though such advice was forthcoming in less than a third of these cases in both groups. As in other areas of research into handicap, a full study of the impact of siblings with multiple handicaps is called for. In the light of this limited information we can go no further than alerting those who come into contact with families with such members to the possible difficulties the non-handicapped children may face.

With respect to wider community attitudes, it was suggested that two possible dimensions were involved. One dimension related to how understanding members of the community were. Respondents were divided on this, though the balance was tipped somewhat towards lack of understanding as the prevailing attitude. Second was the issue of sympathy or its absence. In general the community was thought to be sympathetic, but there was some ambivalence in community attitudes. While sympathy, tolerance and patience might prevail, lack of understanding could lead to embarrassment in dealing with the person with handicaps and his or her family.

With the increasing presence of people with multiple handicaps in the community, understanding might increase through greater contact. However, the consistent view of respondents on how best attitudes could be changed, was through the younger generation. Thus, contact between non-handicapped school children and their peers with multiple handicaps, as well as direct teaching about mental handicap in ordinary schools, was urged. Fourteen and eight per cent of parents of children and adults respectively proposed the integration of children with mental handicap into mainstream schooling. Public education through the media and advertising was also seen to have its place, though few parents saw these as the prime agents of attitude change.

Conclusion

What Hogg, Lambe *et al.* (1987) clearly show is that the day-to-day and life-time problems that have to be dealt with are not a simple summing up of problems in different areas. Difficulties arising from profound retardation and multiple handicaps cannot be viewed in isolation. For example, a family may encounter problems related to travel resulting from an inability of the person with handicaps to walk. Their son or daughter may also exhibit behaviour problems. The presence of such problems when the family are travelling will exacerbate the difficulties of coping with shopping, leisure, or whatever the specific purpose of the trip may be. This state of affairs will influence the attitudes of those in the community who encounter the family and may condition the activities and experiences of siblings. This compounding of effects may in turn lead to increased stress within the family with further detrimental consequences.

Improvement of any key element in this complex chain of events will have wide-ranging benefits that go beyond the single change. Thus reduction or elimination of a behaviour problem could radically affect a family's experience of travel and the attitudes of community and siblings, as well as the overall level of stress experienced by the family.

A variety of professionals have a part to play in providing services which will enable the family to maintain their handicapped member at home. In this review we have described a number of initiatives developed by both the statutory and voluntary sector to realise this objective. Where out-of-family support is required we have seen that both short and long-term fostering are viable options for this group. In addition, there can now be no question that people with profound retardation and multiple handicaps can live in suitably adapted ordinary houses in the community. It is essential, however, that the gap between model provision of the kind that we have described and the frequently inadequate services identified by the MENCAP PRMH Project survey must be closed as a matter of urgency.

Further reading

1. Alaszewski, A., Ong. B. N., Lovett, S., *Croxteth Park Project: Residential care for children who are profoundly mentally handicapped* (Barnado's North West Division, 1986).
2. Dupont, A., 'Medical Results from Registration of Danish Mentally Retarded Persons', in Mittler, P., (ed.) *Frontiers of Knowledge: Volume II* (University Park Press, Baltimore, 1981).
3. Fryers, T., *The Epidemiology of Severe Intellectual Impairment: The dynamics of prevalence* (Academic Press, London, 1984).
4. Hogg, J., Lambe, L., Cowie, J., Coxon, J., *People with Profound Retardation and Multiple Handicaps Attending Schools or Social Education Centres: An interim report on the needs of their parents, foster parents and relatives* (MENCAP, London, 1987).
5. Hogg, J., Sebba, J., *Profound Retardation and Multiple Impairment: Volume 1, Development and Learning* (Croom Helm, London, 1986).
6. Humphreys, S., Lowe, K., de Paiva, S., *Community Care Workers: Part 1. A Description of the Community Care Worker Service in NIMROD* (The Mental Handicap in Wales – Applied Research Unit, Cardiff, 1986).
7. Jacobson, J. W., Sutton, M. S., Janicki, M. P., 'Demography

and Characteristics of Aging and Aged Mentally Retarded Persons', in Janicki, M. P., Wisniewski, H. M., (eds.) *Aging and Developmental Disabilities* (Brookes, Baltimore, 1985).

8. McCorry, S., *The Birmingham Multi-Handicap Group: Northern Project Report* (Birmingham, 1987).

9. MENCAP Homes Foundation, *The Development of Residential Homes for Mentally Handicapped People* (MENCAP, London, 1985).

10. Office of Population Censuses and Services, *Classification of Occupations and Coding Index* (HMSO, London, 1980).

11. Saxby, H., Felce, D., 'The Maintenance of Client Activity and Staff/Client Interaction in Community Homes for Severely and Profoundly Mentally Handicapped Adults: A two year follow-up' (Paper delivered to the British Association for Behavioural Psychotherapy Annual Conference, University of Manchester, 10/12 July 1986).

12. Sebba, J., 'Assessment of Physical Development, Hearing and Vision that Can Be Used by Educational and Care Staff', in Hogg, J., Raynes, N. V., (eds.) *Assessment in Mental Handicap: A guide to assessment practices, tests and checklists* (Croom Helm, London, 1987).

13. Whelan, E., Speake, B., 'A National Survey of Day Provision in England and Wales for Mentally Handicapped Adults with Special Needs: Final report to the Department of Health and Social Security' (University of Manchester, Manchester, 1985).

14. Wolfarth, P., Dodson, L., Dixon, N., Kendall, A., Hardy, J., *Professional Foster Care for Mentally Handicapped Children: The first six placements* (Barnardo's, London, 1985).

CHAPTER 12
Behavioural problems

Dr A. Holland
*Senior Lecturer and Honorary Consultant Psychiatrist, Bethlem
Royal Hospital*

The development of behavioural problems in people who have a
learning disability and who may be mentally handicapped presents
as a problem for society, and the consequences can be serious not
only for the person concerned, but also for his or her family. These
may well extend beyond the existence of the problem behaviour
itself, and the individual's life may become increasingly restricted.
The understandable desperation felt by all concerned may give rise
to a vicious circle of events, more difficulties causing more restrictions and yet further difficulties.

People who are mentally handicapped have difficulty with certain aspects of learning. This may be obvious in the case of people
with more severe impairments who have had great difficulty
learning basic self-care skills. In addition, the development of
language may be very slow and therefore following instructions or
making needs known can be particularly difficult. The causes of the
difficulties are multiple and may be affected by social factors or by
problems such as undetected hearing impairment. The possibility
that a child will have a mental handicap may be recognised at, or
shortly after, birth if he or she has been born with a well-recognised
disorder, known to be associated with learning disabilities. Where
this is not the case, the problem becomes apparent when it is
noticed that the child is slower than usual in his or her development, or requires special help at school. In such disorders as autism
the pattern of development may be abnormal and delayed language
development, together with a history of an absence of normal
childhood play, and often the presence of ritualistic behaviour, are
characteristic. In addition, disorders known to be associated with
mental handicap may also be associated with sensory impairments
or physical abnormalities, the resultant disabilities in turn having an
effect on the person's ability to learn and develop. Looking beyond
these specific problems it is important to appreciate that people
who have similar handicaps may have very little else in common

with one another. Each person is a unique individual: personalities vary, as do interests, experiences and family backgrounds. It is within this context that the occurrence of behavioural problems has to be understood.

The nature of behavioural problems

Referring to something as a 'behavioural problem' neither suggests a cause nor a specific treatment. It is a descriptive term for a particular type of behaviour and does not imply a moral judgment, but rather a recognition that this behaviour is causing distress and as such is contributing to a deterioration in the person's quality of life. The range of problems encountered can be enormous and can include over-activity, aggressive or destructive behaviour, self-injury, noisiness and many others. Some problem behaviours occur at specific times or in specific settings: at meal times, during the night, at school or in a work setting, for example. In some cases, no such link is apparent. The problem may be of recent onset or it may have been present in varying degrees for many years, and other factors such as a change of accommodation or illness in a parent can be the catalyst that leads to the recognition of the problem.

The theoretical backgrounds to understanding behavioural problems fall into two broad groups. A particular behaviour can be seen as bizarre and understandable in terms of 'illness', or the behaviour can be seen to have a 'function'. In the latter case the behaviour has an understandable meaning and results in a particular consequence for the person concerned. It may, for example, bring comfort, or result in the person being left alone or given a drink. Such disparate theories clearly have very different implications for treatment and therefore proper assessment is crucial in deciding the likely explanation of the behaviour in each individual case. Both theoretical frameworks may be important in an individual case, and the reason for continuing a particular behaviour may be quite different from what initiated it.

Assessment of behavioural problems

Behavioural problems in their most severe forms may require a quick response because of the nature of the behaviour, but a proper assessment is essential. The aim of such an assessment is to be able to form a hypothesis regarding the cause of the behavioural problem so that a treatment plan can be established.

Assessment is essentially a two-stage procedure. The first stage is the collection of basic background information. The person whose behaviour is the cause of concern may be able to contribute to this, along with family and care staff. The purpose is to obtain information regarding the cause and degree of mental handicap and the nature of the behavioural problem; in particular, whether it is

Community care and some special groups

lifelong or of recent onset, and whether it occurs at specific times or places. It is important to ask about changes in other areas, for example, loss of abilities, changes in mood and, particularly with adults, evidence of abnormalities of their mental state. This initial information gathering may be sufficient to form an hypothesis about the cause of the behavioural problem. Frequently, however, it is necessary to carry out a more detailed analysis. Stage two of the assessment may involve direct observation, with record-keeping of the frequency of the behaviour and its possible antecedents and consequences. This type of detailed observation of the behaviour, or 'functional analysis', is often referred to as ABC record-keeping, the letters standing for the words 'Antecedent, Behaviour, Consequences'. Such observations try to identify patterns which may be occurring before the onset of the identified behavioural problem, and discover the consequences of the behaviour. For example, self-injurious behaviour may be seen as a means of gaining attention, or as a means of avoiding having to do something else which the person concerned does not like. With these examples the treatment approaches would be very different. Only careful observation can help identify the explanation relevant to a particular case. Having made such an observation, then alternative strategies can be designed to help modify the behaviour.

Increasingly it is recognised that additional factors, referred to as 'setting events', may also be contributing to the occurrence of problem behaviours. Such events are more general factors, individual or environmental, which increase the likelihood of a particular behaviour occurring. An example would be the presence of a bare and unstimulating environment or, at the other extreme, an environment which provides no privacy and is noisy and chaotic. The mood of the person might also be a contributory factor: depression might lower the threshold for the development of behavioural problems. In these situations, antecedent events which normally would not act as a trigger for a particular behaviour may well do so.

Record-keeping

The value of record-keeping depends upon the method producing an accurate record of the behaviour, yet being simple enough for everyone involved to use and understand. In cases where the person is living at home this may not be such a problem, but in hostels or other staffed accommodation it is particularly important. The initial step is to agree upon a definition of the behaviour or behaviours which are a problem (target behaviours). Secondly, the particular aspects of the behaviour, such as its frequency, and possibly the times when it occurs, its nature and antecedents and consequences may all need to be recorded. A simple chart with a column for each is usually sufficient, stating the date, time and so on. To encourage people to keep such records a key worker, or parent, or the person themselves, should transfer basic information into graph form so that variation over time, and the effects of a treatment package, can be easily assessed. Proper and useful record-keeping is a skill, as the observations need to be precise and reliable.

Causes of behavioural problems

An understanding of the cause of a particular behavioural problem requires both a broad theoretical understanding of such problems and the ability to assess the information available in each individual case. There may not be a single cause or explanation of the behaviour, and furthermore, the factors maintaining the behaviour may be different and the behaviour more frequent in some settings than in others. In arriving at a conclusion about the cause of a behavioural problem, three broad headings should be considered as follows:

1. Developmental factors

Temper tantrums are a normal part of development and their absence is abnormal. Children may scream, throw themselves on the ground, break things and so on. This may be a specific response to being told they could not do or have something, or there may be no apparent reason. Tantrums may occur more frequently when a child is tired or hungry or in the context of competition with other siblings. This type of behaviour, although often distressing, is usually understandable, and managing it requires a consistent approach: not giving in, followed later by giving the child some comfort once the temper has subsided. The example of temper tantrums illustrates the important principle that a particular behaviour may have a cause and a consequence. The child may have learnt to use tantrums to get a reward of some sort: sweets or attention, for example. A child who is mentally handicapped may have the additional problem of poor language development and may therefore be less able to express his or her needs. The resources the child has may be more limited and therefore the child may more easily be precipitated into a temper tantrum. With the continuing development of the nervous system as the child is growing, he or she is increasingly able to control outbursts of temper and learn more appropriate and acceptable means of gaining attention or whatever else is desired.

2. Functional/environmental factors

An assessment of the cause of a particular behavioural problem has to attempt to answer several different questions. It is asking: Why has this behaviour started at this point in this person's life? Why does it occur in this particular form and why at these particular times? Changes in circumstances – for example, a change of accommodation – bereavement, boredom, lack of companionship may all be important. In these circumstances, a pattern to the behaviour may emerge. It can be seen to occur at a particular time, and perhaps more often in a particular place, and it usually results in some particular response from others. Proper documentation is crucial in order to arrive at these sorts of conclusion. Such behaviour should not necessarily be seen as wilful 'attention seeking' but rather as a method developed by the individual to communicate his or her needs. This may be an effective, albeit limited, form of communication, but in other ways it is very inappropriate, can cause enormous disruption to everyone and may even be a possible risk to the individual.

3. Psychiatric and individual factors

People who are mentally handicapped may be particularly prone to both physical illnesses and psychiatric disorders. Visual impairment and deafness, both developing insidiously over time, and possibly presenting in the form of behavioural change, are more common in people with Down's Syndrome and in other much rarer genetic disorders. Epilepsy occurs more frequently in people who are mentally handicapped. Poor control of the fits or, conversely, the excessive use of several anti-convulsant drugs, may contribute to behavioural problems. More severely handicapped people may not be able to describe or easily locate pain. Toothache, for example, might be a factor in the onset of self-injurious behaviour to the face. The development of a psychiatric illness in someone who is also mentally handicapped is frequently missed and this too may present as a change in behaviour. The diagnosis relies on careful and sensitive questioning of the person about their mood and strange experiences they may be having: hearing voices, for example, or believing that people are interfering with their brain or bodies. Staff close to the person may have heard the person complaining of these types of abnormal experience. Frequently this is accompanied by a deterioration in the person's general abilities. They may become very restless, or just withdrawn and mute. In the case of depression, sleep is usually disturbed and the person's appetite deteriorates, as does their ability to concentrate. There may be a consistent variation throughout the day, with the mornings usually being the worse time. Manic or hypomanic illnesses are often part of an illness which combines swings of mood in both directions (manic-depressive illness or affective disorder). Mood swings may be triggered by some life-change but then may take on a life of their own and present as a persistent and serious change in mood and behaviour, and may often be accompanied by marked slowing down, agitation or, in the case of mania, over-excitability and irritability. It is important to identify both physical and psychiatric disorders as these are amenable to treatment.

Management of behavioural problems

Good management will be guided by a thorough knowledge of the person and his or her circumstances, and by proper observation. This process of observation in itself can sometimes, in some indeterminate way, help bring the behaviour under control. It gives the parents or care staff a sense that they are beginning to get to grips with the problem, and the person with the behavioural problem can begin to control the behaviour as the responses of those around them are more consistent and positive. It is not possible to describe treatment in detail but any plan of treatment must address the following questions: Why did the behaviour start at this point in time? Is there a characteristic pattern to the frequency and onset of the behaviour? And is the response of others helping to maintain the behaviour? Proper observation will help answer these questions. Treatment is directed at tackling possible underlying causative or contributory factors such as sensory impairments, epilepsy or psychiatric illness. The next step, if appropriate, is to develop strategies to modify the environment, and to agree on an appropriate and consistent response when the behaviour does occur. Any assessment should look at 'good' as well as 'bad' behaviours. Positively rewarding the former, and ignoring the latter, can be a powerful way to bring about the necessary change.

Any management plan decided upon will be influenced by the seriousness of the behaviour. It may be possible to ignore noisy behaviour but not severe self-injurious behaviour. If, however, after the assessment the hypothesis is that a particular behaviour does have a function, then the management will be one of several possible approaches, depending on the exact circumstances. For example, the environment may be a strong determinant of the behaviour and if altered appropriately the frequency of the behaviour may diminish. Alternatively, the behaviour may be a method to obtain staff attention. New, more appropriate, strategies might be taught and the reason for the need for inappropriate behaviour reduced. Ignoring the difficult behaviour and only responding positively at times of appropriate behaviour may give lead to a reduction of the former and an increase in the latter types of behaviour.

An essential feature of all treatment plans should be proper and reliable record-keeping of the behaviour. A two-week baseline measure of the behaviour, its nature and frequency, can be invaluable so that any treatment or management plan can easily be assessed. A particular management package may be wrong and only proper observation can assess this.

Behaviour associated with specific disorders

The causes of mental handicap are multiple and it is not possible to know all of them or the details of every rare disorder. It is, however, important to consider the possibility that a particular behaviour is characteristic of a particular syndrome. If this is the case there may be specific treatments, or at least a body of useful knowledge about how this type of problem might be tackled.

Two examples of this are the Lesch-Nyan Syndrome, a rare disorder affecting males only and associated with severe self-injurious behaviour, and the Prader-Willi Syndrome, associated with excessive eating and resultant obesity. Similarly, specific handicapping disorders may be associated with secondary problems which may present initially as changes in behaviour. An example of this is that of Down's Syndrome. People born with this disorder are prone to a variety of problems as they grow older, particularly impaired vision and hearing, and in middle age they may develop a dementing illness called Alzheimer's disease. These problems may give rise to a change in behaviour, for example, stubbornness, aggressiveness or increasing self-neglect and social withdrawal.

A diagnosis of the cause of the handicap may also be important as it may have implications in terms of that person's sociability and pattern of handicap. People who, for a number of reasons, may have the features of autism not only have delayed language development but also have a marked impairment of social functioning. They frequently find change particularly difficult to deal with and dislike being pressurised into taking part in social activities. Behavioural problems may develop because of a change in staff or routine which is easily coped with by others but not by the person who is autistic. The change which has taken place may not be perceived by other people and may be, for example, a minor change in the position of a piece of furniture or in the daily routine.

Conclusions

The occurrence of behavioural difficulties in people with learning disabilities can have a major effect on the person concerned, their families and their care staff. The causes of such problems are multiple and can often only be established as a result of careful observation and the collection of information about the cause of the handicap, the circumstances before and after each episode of behavioural disturbance, and other individual and environmental information. The problem may be primarily related to the developmental level of the person, and under these circumstances appropriate and consistent management of each episode may give rise to a reduction in the problem behaviour. In other cases, additional factors may be, or may once have been, contributing to the development and the maintenance of the problem.

The management of behavioural problems depends on being able to recognise what factors are important and then developing a strategy to change them. This may be the use of a consistent approach by all concerned with the management of the behaviour, or it may require the treatment of other problems such as psychiatric illness, epilepsy or the correction of a visual or hearing impairment. The problem may be related to boredom, lack of occupation or sexual concerns. As treatments and different methods of management are tried, their effects should be monitored by careful observation and record-keeping. Many problems may diminish using a logical approach, but if behavioural problems persist then further help should be obtained from the specialists working within the psychiatric or mental handicap services.

Behavioural problems should not be accepted as inevitable or unalterable. However, neither should a person who has a learning disability be expected to be perfect. The skill is to allow the individual concerned to retain some responsibility for their life and to maintain their dignity, yet to help them bring their inappropriate behaviour back under control.

Further reading

1. Corbett, J. A., 'Psychiatry and Mental Retardation', *Scientific Studies in Mental Retardation*, Editors: Dobbing, J., Clarke, A. D. B., Corbett, J. A., Hogg, J., Robinson, R. O., (Royal Society of Medicine, London, 1984).
2. Kiernan, C., 'Behaviour Modification', *Mental Deficiency: The Changing Outlook*, Editors: Clarke, A. M., Clarke, A. D. B., Berg, J. M., (Methuen and Co. Ltd, London, 1985).
3. Murphy, G., 'Direct Observation as an Assessment Tool in Functional Analysis and Treatment', *Assessment in Mental Handicap: A Guide to Assessment Practices, Tests and Checklists*, Editors: Hogg, J., Raynes, N., (Croom Helm, London, 1987).

CHAPTER 13

Ageing and mental handicap

Dr James Hogg, Steve Moss and Diane Cooke
*Reader and Deputy Director; Research Fellow and Research
Assistant, Hester Adrian Research Centre, University of Manchester*

That we live in an ageing society is by now a piece of information familiar to most people. 'Welcome to the global old folks' home!' writes Pearce (1987) drawing attention to the phenomenon of an ageing world but at the same time pointing out just how inaccurate demographers can be in making exact predictions. He cites Enid Charles as arguing that after the massive losses of World War I there would be a continually falling birth rate that would leave England and Wales with a population of 10 million in the early twenty-first century!

With respect to people with mental handicap we must exercise some caution when trying to establish how many will survive into the later decades, but must note that the same general trends as may be anticipated in the wider population will almost certainly occur, and for basically the same reasons. A critical determinant of increasing longevity is the improving quality of medical care and people with mental handicap have undoubtedly benefited, as have their non-handicapped peers. Indeed, for some individuals with mental handicap who are particularly prone to certain illnesses, these medical advances have had an even greater impact. Advances in perinatal care have resulted in a much greater proportion of impaired children surviving the first year of life, so that Fryers (1984) is able to report a current death rate of only 10 per cent among children with Down's syndrome compared with 50 per cent in earlier studies (Carter, 1958; Hall, 1964; Oster, 1953; Record and Smith, 1955). Among adults, a similar decline has been observed as former major causes of death have been eradicated or controlled. Tuberculosis, pneumonia and influenza were responsible for 50 to 60 per cent of deaths among people with severe mental handicap, a rate 13 times greater than for the general population (Conley, 1973). The change can be dramatically illustrated through a direct comparison of two studies undertaken 40 years apart. Dayton *et al.* (1932) found 28 per cent of the people alive at 10 years survived to

60. Balakrishnan and Wolf (1976) report an equivalent figure of 46 per cent.

Not all conditions giving rise to mental handicap follow the trend to the same degree. Exact estimates of numbers of people over a given age now and at future dates are extremely difficult to establish.

Characteristics

Research in the field of mental handicap has concentrated over-whelmingly on children and to a lesser extent on young adults. There is a dearth of information on even the most basic aspects of health, mental state and adaptive functioning in older individuals. Such information as exists is of some relevance to those providing services in the community for people with mental handicap as they age. Elsewhere we have provided a detailed review of the available literature and identified some of the methodological and substantive issues that need to be addressed (Hogg, Moss and Cooke, 1988). Here we will note some of the main conclusions drawn in that review.

In line with Jacobson, Sutton and Janicki (1985), our own examination of the available literature suggested that the health status of older people with mental handicap is broadly comparable to that of the wider population. Where a condition is more evident among people with mental handicap, then it typically reflects a chronic physical condition that predates the onset of ageing. Comparing the psychiatric problems of elderly people with and without mental handicap is made difficult by the contrasting life-styles of the two populations and by the well-established fact that the two major conditions associated with ageing, depression and dementia, often go undetected in older people in the general population. Elderly people with mental handicap show even lower referral rates than their non-handicapped peers, though in a recent paper Day (1987) has indicated that the prevalence of age-related psychiatric conditions in people with and without mental handicap do not differ. In reality a definitive statement awaits fuller psychiatric investigations which in turn will necessitate the development of diagnostic criteria applicable to individuals with widely differing life-styles and levels of ability.

In older people with mental handicap the diagnosis of dementia is a particularly sensitive issue as a variety of conditions can mimic the symptoms of this condition. In addition, because of reduced communicative abilities in people with mental handicap the close observation of family and friends can be of great assistance to the psychiatrist. More generally, it is important for family and carers to be aware that older people with mental handicap *can* suffer from psychiatric disorders and that changes in day-to-day functioning can be important indicators of the development of such conditions. Referral to a psychiatrist then becomes imperative.

One specific condition on which more information can be provided is the hypothesised link between Down's syndrome and the condition of presenile dementia known as Alzheimer's disease. Pathological changes in the brain associated with this disease have undoubtedly been demonstrated in numerous post-mortem studies of people with Down's syndrome. Nevertheless, occurrence of these signs does not necessarily mean the person has actually displayed the symptoms of Alzheimer's disease and it is quite incorrect to suggest that all people with Down's syndrome living into their third, fourth or fifth decade will inevitably display the condition.

Owens, Dawson and Losin (1971) studied two groups of Down's syndrome residents at a state hospital in California. One group consisted of residents over 35; the other aged from 20 to 25. Measures were taken of the functioning of the frontal and parietal lobes, and a questionnaire was devised to test memory, orientation, agnosia, and apraxia. Following examination of all members of the older sample it was concluded that *none* of them could be unequivocally classified as suffering from dementia. Reid and Aungle (1974) assessed 155 hospital residents over 45 years of age for clinical evidence of dementia. Eight of these 155 residents had Down's syndrome. The authors found eleven of the group to be suffering from dementia, giving an overall prevalence rate of 7.1 per cent. Of the 155 residents, 22 were aged 65 or over, and three of these 22 were dementing, giving a prevalance rate of 13.6 per cent for this age group. Two of the eight with Down's syndrome were included in the group of 11 suffering from dementia. This represents a prevalence rate of 25 per cent compared with six per cent of the people without Down's syndrome. Despite this apparently large differential, it must be borne in mind that the numbers are too small to provide a reliable estimate.

Traditionally, ageing in the general population has been associated with both intellectual and physical decline. More specifically, such decline has been viewed as biomedical in origin – unavoidable and irreversible. Since the early 1970s, however, this view has been extensively challenged. First, a number of studies have shown that even serious decline in a variety of communicative and adaptive functions is often determined by disadvantaging aspects of the social and physical environment in which the older person finds him or herself. Suitable intervention can often lead to restoration of function with consequent improvements in the quality of an individual's life. Second, the popular belief that serious intellectual decline inevitably occurs with age requires qualification. Marked decline in intellectual function in the absence of organic causes is typically *not* found until after the age of 70 years. However, what decline occurs does not affect all aspects of intellectual functioning. Typically verbal ability will remain high, representing as it does the consolidation or 'crystallised' intelligence that a person has acquired throughout her or his lifetime through decades of social experience. In contrast, what has been called 'fluid' intelligence, i.e., the intellectual processes that deal with the understanding of unfamiliar material, does show some decline in the later years. This differential decline in verbal (or crystallised) intelligence, and performance (or fluid intelligence) has been referred to as the classic ageing pattern. Nevertheless, one eminent US worker, Schaie (1983) argues that even at 81, less than half of all individuals in his own study showed reliable changes in the previous seven years.

Comparable evidence on people with mental handicap is more limited than from the non-handicapped population. We do know, however, that throughout most of their life-span, from young adulthood to the 60s, improvements in intellectual functioning typically occur (Fisher and Zeaman, 1970). Where decrements do occur, they come well into later life. Research on differential changes in verbal and performance abilities is, however, lacking in the population of people with mental handicap. A further important point that must be noted is that most studies of the growth of intelligence in people with mental handicap have taken place on individuals living in large institutions which are known to be less than optimal with respect to intellectual development. If we bear in mind the point made above regarding the impact of the environment on the ageing person, then we might anticipate that an even more optimistic picture of intellectual growth would emerge if studies were conducted on people living in the community as well as those already studied in institutions.

Moving on from the somewhat abstract concept of intelligence, we can also ask how ageing people with mental handicap cope with the demands of the real world through adaptive or functional behaviour. What is the course of development in these areas as people with mental handicap get older? Again, studies have typically been conducted on people living in large institutions. Nihira (1976) employed the American Association on Mental Deficiency Adaptive Behavior Scales to answer this question. Here a general picture emerges of individuals with mental handicap gaining in self-sufficiency until well into their 40s, with only small decrements occurring after 50 in people who are borderline, mildly or moderately mentally handicapped. Those who were severely or profoundly mentally handicapped continue to make progress throughout their life-span.

Bear in mind that these reported gains have been observed in depriving, institutional environments in which educational or social programmes will have been lacking. We must once again ask, what potential for life-span development would be realised by all people with mental handicap if they led their lives in more stimulating circumstances? Though research is generally limited, it is not unreasonable to suggest that, as in the case of their non-handicapped peers, people with mental handicap can develop throughout most of their lives, and that the process of ageing does not need to be an additional handicap that curtails their opportunities.

We have, then, a population of people with mental handicap of whom a significant proportion will reach old age with no greater likelihood of physical or mental illness than their peers who are not mentally handicapped. They will also have the same opportunity to develop personally, socially and with respect to their competence in a variety of areas of life. For others, life expectancy will remain lower than average, albeit continuing to increase as medical provision leads to improvements in their health, particularly in the case of people with Down's syndrome, while life will be even more curtailed for some individuals with profound retardation and multiple physical, sensory and health impairments.

Ageing and transition

The consequences of ageing for people with mental handicap is, then, a generally positive one. There is nothing in the admittedly limited information we have reviewed that would suggest that there is any justification for discriminating against such people with respect to their having an equal opportunity to come to live in local neighbourhoods or to continue their lives there. This distinction is an important one as we are looking at two populations of people, those in the long-stay hospitals and those living in the community at present with family, friends or in some form of local authority provision. In some hospitals more than half of the residents will be over 50 years of age, with several well into their 90s; in the community, the largest single group of carers of adults with mental handicap are parents. One estimate suggests 60,000 adults living with their families (DHSS, 1971), 10,000 of these with parents who are over 70. The process of caring for these two populations in the community involves a variety of common elements and contrasts with which we deal below. First, however, we must draw a distinction that will help us to focus on these similarities and differences.

Elsewhere (Hogg, Moss and Cooke, 1988) it has been suggested that the process of ageing is essentially one of continual change. The gradual transitions involved in ageing related to general physical well-being and changing competence can be viewed as progressive, i.e, they take place over time and are not obviously related to specific happenings. In contrast, some change is specifically related to identifiable events. The transition from one residence to another or from active engagement in work to the opportunity to engage in leisure pursuits is clearly marked and can and does occur at a specific time on a given day.

With respect to progressive transitions, both hospital-based and community-based people with mental handicap will show gradual changes in functional and adaptive abilities as described in our introduction. One concomitant of such changes will be that they will have need of a variety of services to facilitate positive change and cope with developing difficulties. These changes do not take place in a vacuum, however, and we would expect the differing physical and social environments in which the two groups live to have contrasting effects. With regard to event-related changes, movement from hospital to community and family home to community involve differing forms of initial adjustment, though in the longer term the needs of individuals for services will not necessarily differ. Our subsequent discussion, therefore, needs to consider both progressive change and demand for services in the community and the nature of specific transitions and their consequences for older people with mental handicap. It should be added, however, that for any individual, life will be made up of both forms of change and that they will interact to condition the sum total of the person's ageing experience. Both availability of information and space preclude any consideration of all the permutations that contrasted residential conditions and characteristic of people with mental handicap could generate. We will therefore focus on three broad areas of interest before concluding with a general consideration of community provision:

1. Life in the parental home, and after.
2. Relocation from hospitals into ordinary urban neighbourhoods.
3. The process of adjustment as more able people age in the community.

Life in the parental home, and after

By far the single largest group of carers of adults with mental handicap living in the community are parents. Against the background of both the demographic and service changes we have described above, this number will almost certainly continue to increase. This state of affairs raises two central issues. The first relates to the contemporary situation as families cope on a day-to-day and year-to-year basis with their ageing sons and daughters. The second concern is preparation for the future as parents themselves age, and eventually die, with inevitable consequences for the practicality of maintaining their son or daughter at home.

Support for the family

In our own interviews with service providers it has been reported that older families with a son or daughter living at home do not present a consistent problem to services. Such families have learnt to cope over many years, often without adequate professional input when it was most needed. Studies in Wales by Grant (1985; 1986) have shown that there is an enormous range and great variation in the material and social resources on which these carers can draw. However, the lifelong care at home of people with mental handicap is typically undertaken by women. For them is the primary responsibility of personal care, bathing and dressing, even when advanced in years themselves. Even when available to help through retirement or unemployment, fathers are much less frequently involved in these activities. What leads parents, particularly mothers, to be so self-sufficient in these caring activities, often avoiding dependency on professionals and friends and neighbours alike?

Grant has suggested six main reasons as follow:

1. Parents wish to maintain their own independence.
2. For many parents the problem is not a problem. They have developed well-established routines for managing the needs of their sons and daughters and could often anticipate and avoid potential problems. Thus they reject any suggestion that caring is unduly intrusive in their lives.
3. Parents often wish to avoid experiencing unsympathetic attitudes and achieve this by maintaining their son or daughter in the family home and reducing contact with the outside world.
4. Many parents believe that special knowledge and understanding is needed to look after their son or daughter, and that they above all have this requisite knowledge.
5. Grant draws a distinction between caring for and caring about their son or daughter. They see it as their role to care for their off-spring, asking only for moral support, i.e., demonstrations of caring for their son or daughter, from others.
6. To accept support from friends or neighbours implies some kind of indebtedness and therefore some degree of dependency on them. This is a situation best avoided by only drawing on such help on an intermittent basis.

Indeed, research has shown that with respect to other family members, notably the mental handicapped individual's brothers and sisters, and friends and neighbours, support for the family is limited. This does not mean that these sources of support are uncaring or unsympathetic, only that the parents themselves choose to cope with minimum demands on those outside the home.

Given the ability of parents over many decades to successfully maintain their son or daughter in the family home, what are the rewards and stresses of such care? Richardson and Ritchie (1986) have explored this question in interviews with parents. They note that there are two complex sets of emotional responses. On the one hand, there is a very positive side arising from a strong parental bond and the pleasure in having a loved child at home. On the other, there is a negative side, arising from the stress on a family of coping with a member with a handicap. These authors believe that the strength of the conflicting responses depends largely on the nature of the son's or daughter's handicap *and* the amount of support parents receive. Both positive and negative experiences will be involved for most families. Wertheimer (1981) contrasts the negative view of mental handicap with the positive picture that emerges of warm family relations between parents and their son or daughter, but notes that this every intimacy can accentuate problems of separation when the parents can no longer cope.

Preparing for the future

In the many studies that have now been undertaken on how ageing families provide for their adult son or daughter, a recurrent theme and, indeed, primary concern is: 'What will happen to my son or daughter when we can no longer cope?' As one parent commented: 'It is something that I think about every day of my life.' Ritchie and Richardson suggest that there are three primary attitudes: avoidance, ambivalence and the active search for future accommodation. Their own study indicates that the most likely attitudes are avoidance and ambivalence, with only a minority of families making preparatory plans. They quote one parent as stating: 'We just live from day to day, you know, and don't look too far into the future. One year is much like another year . . . I think if with something like this you were to look too much in the future, and dwell on it too much, then I think you would get despondent.' Our own studies in Manchester have clearly confirmed this state of affairs (Cooke, 1987).

This situation raises numerous questions. Given the general lack of preparation, have families even discussed that issue with other people? Typically, discussion has taken place, but usually only within the family. Social workers report that frequently, when they raise the issue of the future, parents often refuse to pursue the topic. Notably, parents rarely discuss future plans with the person they will most affect, i.e., their mentally handicapped son or daughter.

When consideration is given to future plans, what form do these take? A substantial number of parents will look towards other family menbers for support, notably their son's or daughter's siblings. In some cases siblings will have accepted this responsibility, but in others the parents are making an assumption about future arrangements that has never been fully discussed and about which siblings have not given a formal undertaking. Many families will, however, accept the need for statutory residential provision. Here the main criteria of acceptability are, first, a guarantee of permanence, i.e., that their son or daughter will be able to live in that accommodation for the rest of their lives, and second, homeliness. These requirements of permanence and homeliness can, of course, lead to a preference for a variety of different forms of accommodation, from small groups of people living in ordinary housing, to village communities.

Most studies are in agreement, however, that despite these preliminary discussions on future plans, and some conception of what would be desirable, only small percentages of people have actually made formal plans and begun the process of 'letting go' prior to their own death or incapacity. It is easy from what we have reported earlier to understand why this situation pertains. The parents *are* coping and in many respects the situation is an emotionally rewarding one. But what of the son or daughter who will eventually have to cope with the crisis of relocation when his or her parents can no longer cope? This situation will be exacerbated because not only may the son or daughter have to cope with a move to unfamiliar accommodation for which they have not been prepared, but also may have to deal with the loss of a loved parent. It is clear that many people with mental handicap suffer from this dual blow, and that professional staff are often insensitive to their need for emotional support and understanding. Elsewhere we have drawn attention to the relevant literature on bereavement with respect to ways with which the experience may most constructively be dealt (Hogg, Moss and Cooke, 1988).

Finally, as with the rest of the population, people with mental handicap will benefit from adequate legal provision for the future as they and their parents age. Typically a significant majority of families will have failed in this respect (see Warren and Mulcahey, 1984, and Cooke, 1987). Advice from relevant professionals in conjunction with solicitors has a vital role to play in enabling the person with mental handicap to receive resources that can be critical to a successful life in the community. Though now requiring some up-dating, Sanctuary's (1984) exemplary book is essential reading on this subject, while the British Institute of Mental Handicap have produced a bibliography on this subject. In addition the Royal Society for Mentally Handicapped Children and Adults have their own legal department and advisory service.

From institution to the wider community

Implicit in the preceding discussion is the fact that the transition from family home to ordinary housing in the neighbourhood or town *can* be effected prior to a crisis in which the possibility of successful adjustment is endangered. This is dependent upon preparation of the person with mental handicap, the family, and on society making available suitable accommodation and services. The opportunity for similar preparation is clearly available to those who are implementing the care in the community initiative with respect to hospital closure. As yet this has not had to be effected in crisis conditions as the run-down of hospitals is occurring with characteristic British gradualism.

In considering the relocation of older people with mental handicap, the question is often raised as to whether it would not be preferable to let them remain in such institutions rather than subject them to the shock of the difficult transition to life in the wider community, a transition that may well have quite adverse consequences for their physical and psychological well-being. Second, what is the fate of people with mental handicap who from young adulthood or the middle years live, and grow older, in the community? Do the associated pressures of an intellectual disability and the concomitants of ageing make this a difficult or even impossible way of life?

Although lip-service is paid to treating older people with mental handicap on an equal basis to their younger peers, we have a strong impression that the former are often discriminated against when consideration is given to moving them from various forms of congregate care to smaller community units or homes. Often they are the last to be considered for relocation, and in some instances this policy is made explicit. The rationale for delay or refusal in moving them usually relates to the assumption that they would suffer from what has been called 'relocation trauma'.

In the wider literature on relocation trauma in older people without mental handicap it is clear that there are many factors that have to be taken into account in evaluating research on this subject. With respect to the most undesirable outcome of relocation, it is clear that there are as many studies showing increased mortality following a move as there are those showing a decrease. Similarly, improvements in health following relocation have been reported frequently in the literature. Factors which affect the outcome relate to the nature of the move itself. A move from one's own home to a larger institution is obviously qualitatively very different from a move from one homely environment to another. Second, whether the move is voluntary or enforced may have an important effect with respect to the outcome, though as yet there is no clear research to support this proposition.

In general, studies of relocation among people with mental handicap have not shown any increase in mortality. At a behavioural level Landesman-Dwyer (1982) showed no differences between older and younger residents who were moved from a large institutional setting into remodelled residential units – except, perhaps like the rest of us, the older folk sleep more! Similarly, Heller (1982) presents evidence on residents over 50 years of age who were transferred from a large institution to smaller residences. Six months later this older group of people showed no indication of adverse effects of the transfer, while 30 months later older and younger individuals showed the same degree of behavioural adaptation to the community.

The generally positive outcomes we have described should not be taken as indicating that the transition involved in making the adjustment to relocation is necessarily an easy one – only that when suitably dealt with it can be achieved even by older people with mental handicap. It is obviously important that care is taken in preparing the person for the change and familiarising them with the new setting in which they are going to live. In addition, support from service providers, friends and family must minimise the stress that inevitably comes in coping with a new set of demands. It is of interest to note that in one of the few findings in which relocation led to a marked increase in mortality, the people involved had profound retardation and were possibly unable to cope with the stress through their own lack of coping mechanisms. However, studies in the UK are now plentiful with respect to relocation of people with profound retardation, and successful adjustment and gains in adaptive behaviour are typically reported.

Age itself, then, should not be regarded as a bar to older people with mental handicap availing themselves of the changing pattern of services that the movement to community living is opening up. With careful preparation and subsequent support, the benefits of living in ordinary locations and participating in the life of the community can be enjoyed, and may embrace work and leisure activities, as well as participating in the spiritual life of the community in their chosen religious organisations.

We can, however, embrace a wider span by considering the lives of people who have spent several decades in the community, not in the parental home or with siblings, but living relatively independently. At this point in the history of mental handicap and society, such people are most likely to be mildly or moderately mentally handicapped, and indeed, the information we have is inevitably limited to a small number of significant studies. Perhaps the key concept, apart from the psychological resources of the people themselves, is that of informal support networks. Leaving to one side family support, which will be dealt with in the next section, we are here talking about the support of friends, neighbours and acquaintances. To consider this issue we will examine one important group of studies undertaken by Edgerton in the USA and one of the few such studies offering a longitudinal perspective.

In 1967 Edgerton published 'The Cloak of Competence: Stigma

in the Lives of the Mentally Retarded', an ethnographic study of 48 residents of a large institution who were discharged into the community. Of relatively high IQ (mean=64), these men and women showed broadly successful adaptation to their new life, though Edgerton's research drew attention to the fact that this successful adjustment owed a great deal to non-retarded benefactors rather than to any specific level of skill, attitude or training. He also describes the strategies by which these people attempted to present themselves to the world as 'normal', strategies which often did not actually reflect true competence in that they essentially found ways round problematical situations rather than actually coping with the difficulty.

The situation just described pertained in 1960–61 after the individuals had spent six years in the community. Edgerton and Berkovici (1976) report on a follow-up of traceable people some twelve years later in 1972–73, while Edgerton, Bollonger and Herr (1984) report a further investigation in 1982. In the early 1970s those who could be located were in their mid 40s. In 1982, the comparable mean chronological age was 56 years.

Social competence and independence were judged through a variety of observer ratings such as economic security, relative independence, social participation, absence of antisocial behaviour, employment, sexual-marital adjustment and feelings of stigma. In the 1976 study, the life circumstances in eight individuals were, overall, considered better, 12 the same and ten worse, relative to the 1967 study. There was great diversity in the lives of people *within* each of these groups. One man had indeed initially been among the most competent in the group and had gone from strength to strength, while one woman, 'formerly cloistered, timid and dependent' had begun to venture into the world and assert herself. Nora had initially earned her living as a headless lady at an amusement park, engaging in passing affairs and living partially off welfare. By the early 1970s she was married with three children, working with her husband in a factory and with a pleasant stable home life.

Similar diversity would be found among those who had not successfully adjusted. Robert, of average independence in the original study, was initially employed and sharing an appartment with a homosexual man. In 1972–3 he was 'penniless and hungry with no place to sleep and was apparently an alcoholic as well', surviving by selling his blood. Dorothy was dependent on her first husband in 1960–1, but in her next marriage after his death was not only dependent, but subject to difficulties linked to heroin and her husband's increasing age, with few resources and little hope for the future.

In Edgerton's (1967) study the high dependence on benefactors and concern with stigma that we noted above were critical elements in the social thinking of the individuals studied. While the reasons for the change are not clear, dependence on benefactors and concern with stigma appeared to play a less important role in 1972–3 than it had done earlier. However, with a further 12 years of experience the need for support may well have reduced while in parallel the belief in stigma attaching to oneself would decline. These trends continued throughout the subsequent decade as Edgerton, Bollonger and Herr (1984) reported later.

In 1984 Edgerton, Bollonger and Herr extended the period of study of this group to 20 years of community living noting that their concern was now explicitly with the process of ageing. Again, change in the lives of the individuals was a central concern and ratings indicated that over the past decade one person's life was 'in continuous flux', the lives of five were stable, for four life had deteriorated and for three it had improved. For two the complexity was so great that they defied categorisation. Edgerton *et al.* see the major factors in influencing them to be related to the social and personal resources available to the individuals. With respect to the four people whose lives had worsened, a major loss had been sustained while none had a strong benefactor, a support network or service support.

Decline in health was found in ten individuals both in the 1972–3 and 1982 studies. Of the 30 individuals in the former study one was terminally ill and nine had disabling ailments. No one showed improvements in health since 1960–1. By 1982, ten of the sample of 15 had declined further and all of them realised that this was related to old age. While some used their condition strategically others refused to 'give in'.

Edgerton *et al.* describe with characteristic concinnity the resilience with which most individuals cope with the social and health changes that accompanied ageing in contrast to their dependency:

'There is a central theme to their lives, whether those lives have worsened, improved, or remained very much the same; the theme is hope. With the exception of one woman who was quite depressed, all the rest had an unshakeable optimism; they still had hope that life would be rewarding, or more rewarding than it had been, and they believed that their own actions could help to bring this outcome to pass.'

Edgerton and his colleagues show that their own predictions regarding each individual's degree of success in adjusting to the community was often highly inaccurate even when the person had been in the community for several years. With respect to the prediction of successful community adjustment as people get older, Edgerton and Berkovici (1976) argue that we cannot simply predict on the basis of an individual's characteristics but must also include in the equation such matters as public attitudes, welfare legislation, or employment opportunities which can, in principle, have profound effects on social adjustment, as can differences in residential environments.

Services and the ageing population

We know very little about the way in which service needs change as people with mental handicap grow older in the community. Seltzer, Seltzer and Sherwood (1982) in a US study compared a group of older people with mental handicap (55 years+) with a younger group (18–54 years). Their results suggest that though the older people had a greater need for a variety of services, they actually received fewer than did their younger peers. Certainly we would expect older people with mental handicap to show the increase in need for medical and psychiatric treatment that occurs in the wider population. It is also consistent with the nature of community care that these be provided by the generic services within the District Health Authority. At issue is the adequacy of the physical and mental health screening of people who may be unable to communicate their own condition to others. This is a crucial issue and one which merits careful attention as part of the process of evaluating the success of the community care initiative.

With respect to wider social needs, it was noted in the introduction that well into their later years many people with mental handicap show the potential for continuing development. For a relatively limited number of people aged 50 years or over, paid employment will occupy some of their later years, while for others, continued activity of various kinds will be available in Adult Training Centres. For individuals in both these settings, retirement will be another critical transition in their lives, and one which has been discussed in detail elsewhere (Hogg, Moss and Cooke 1988). Following retirement, and for those who have not been involved in employment and day-service provision, the later years will need to be occupied in such a way that both their own inclinations and preferences are met and their capacity to continue to develop is acknowledged. To meet these objectives both educational and leisure opportunities need to be provided with as much urgency as is the case for younger adults.

Though we know of no systematic survey of the national situation with respect to providing such services for older people with mental handicap, it is clear from the authors' own experiences that provision is highly variable. With respect to education, older people are in some areas involved in colleges of further education, community colleges, and in-house programmes provided by staff and visiting teachers. In other contexts, no such initiative is being attempted and passivity and stagnation are the orders of the day. Leisure provision can also be seen on a dimension that extends from thoughtful and varied active pursuits to passive consumption of television and radio as a virtually full-time occupation. The positive contribution of specialist clubs such as those organised by the Gateway Federation has a widely acknowledged contribution to make in this area. The extent to which changes in provision related to age necessitates revision of on-going programmes, is one of active concern.

With respect to both educational and leisure provision, two further considerations merit comment. First, developing programmes differ with respect to how far they attempt to utilise provision for the wider ageing community. With social integration as the ultimate aim of community care the initiative to involve older people with mental handicap in such provision is of special importance. It would seem inherently undesirable to create yet another segregated population: aged people with mental handicap. Second, the lot of older people in the UK and other Western countries is far from enviable. Material and service shortcoming result in poverty, misery, and even death. Many people with mental handicap have only the most limited resources and any simplistic interpretation of the concept of normalisation would lead them in the direction of the wider population of less-fortunate older people. Wolfensberger (1985) has commented on this situation and urged that special, additional resources are made available to enable older people with mental handicap not just to survive in the community, but to enjoy their later years as a positive and self-enhancing period of their lives. Both our knowledge of these people and the potential offered by an adequately resourced policy of community care could make this apparently idealistic objective a reality.

Further reading

1. Balakrishnan, T. R., Wolf, L. C., 'Life expectancy of mentally retarded persons in Canadian institutions', *American Journal of Mental Deficiency*, vol. 80, (1976), pp.650–62.
2. Carter, C. O., 'A life-table for mongols with the causes of death', *Journal of Mental Deficiency Research*, vol. 2, (1958), pp.64–74.
3. Conley, R. W., *The economics of mental retardation* (Johns Hopkins, Baltimore, 1973).
4. Cooke, D. J., *Older parents and their adult sons and daughters with mental handicap: Home lives and future plans* (Unpublished MSc thesis, University of Manchester, 1987).
5. Day, K., 'The elderly mentally handicapped in hospital: A clinical study, *Journal of Mental Deficiency Research*, (1987), vol. 31, pp.131–46.
6. Dayton, N. A., Doering, C. R., Hilferty, M. M., Maher,

H. C., Dolan, H. H., 'Mortality and expectation of life in mental deficiency in Massachusetts: Analysis of the fourteen year period 1917–1930', *New England Journal of Medicine*, vol. 206, (1932), pp.555–70.

7. Department of Health and Social Security, *Better services for the mentally handicapped* (II(Cmnd 4683), HMSO, 1971).
8. Edgerton, R. B., *The cloak of competence: Stigma in the lives of the mentally retarded* (University of California Press, Berkeley, 1967).
9. Edgerton, R. B., Berkovici, S. M., 'The cloak of competence: Years later', *American Journal of Mental Deficiency*, vol. 80, (1976), pp.485–97.
10. Edgerton, R. B., Bollonger, M., Herr, B., 'The cloak of competence: After two decades', *American Journal of Mental Deficiency*, vol. 88, (1984), pp.345–51.
11. Fisher, M. A., Zeaman, D., 'Growth and decline of retardate intelligence' in Ellis, N. R., (ed.), *International review of research on mental retardation* (vol. 4) (Academic Press, London, 1970).
12. Fryers, T., *The epidemiology of severe intellectual impairment: The dynamics of prevalence* (Academic Press, London, 1984).
13. Grant, G., *Older carers, interdependence and the care of mentally handicapped adults* (University College of North Wales, Bangor, Gwynedd, 1985).
14. Grant, G., *Working Paper No. 41* (Social Policy and Development Centre, University College of North Wales, Bangor, Gwynedd, 1986).
15. Hall, B., 'Mongolism in newborns. A clinical and cytogenic study', *Acta Paediatrica* (Stockholm), Supplement 154, (1964).
16. Heller, T., 'The effects of involuntary residential relocation: A review', *American Journal of Community Psychology*, vol. 10, (1982), pp.471–92.
17. Hogg, J., Moss, S. C., Cooke, D., *Ageing and mental handicap* (Chapman & Hall, London, 1988).
18. Jacobson, J. W., Sutton, M. S., Janicki, M. P., 'Demography and characteristics of ageing and aged mentally retarded persons' in Janicki, M. P., Wisniewski, H. M., (eds.), *Ageing and developmental disabilities: Issues and approaches* (Paul Brookes Publishing, Baltimore, 1985).
19. Landesman-Dwyer, S., *The changing structure and function of institutions: A search for optimal group care environments* (Paper presented at Lake Wilderness conference on Impact of Residential Environments on Retarded Persons, 1982).
20. Nihira, K., 'Dimensions of adaptive behavior in institution-alized mentally retarded children and adults: Developmental perspective', *American Journal of Mental Deficiency*, vol. 81, (1976), pp.215–26.
21. Oster, J., *Mongolism: A clinicogeneological investigation comprising*

526 mongols living on Seeland (Danish Science Press, Copenhagen, 1953).

22. Owens, D., Dawson, J. C., Losin, S., 'Alzheimer's disease in Down's syndrome', *American Journal of Mental Deficiency*, vol. 75, (1971), pp.606–12.
23. Pearce, F., 'Welcome to the Global Old Folks' Home', *New Scientist*, 9 July 1987, pp.32–5.
24. Record, R. G., Smith, A., 'The incidence, mortality, and sex distributions of mongoloid defectives', *British Journal of Preventative Social Medicine*, vol. 9, (1955), pp.10–15.
25. Reid, A. H., Aungle, P. G., 'Dementia in ageing mental defectives: A clinical psychiatric study', *Journal of Mental Deficiency Research*, vol. 18, (1974), pp.15–23.
26. Richardson, A., Ritchie, J., 'Making the break: Parents' views about adults with a mental handicap leaving the parental home' (Kings' Fund Centre, London, 1986).
27. Sanctuary, G., *After I'm gone (What will happen to my handicapped child?)* (Souvenir Press, London, 1984).
28. Schaie, K. W., 'The Seattle longitudinal study: A 21-year exploration of psychometric intelligence in adulthood' in Schaie, K. W., (ed.), *Longitudinal studies of adult psychological development* (The Guilford Press, New York, 1983).
29. Seltzer, M. M., Seltzer, G. B., Sherwood, C. C., 'Comparison of community adjustment of older vs. younger mentally retarded adults', *American Journal of Mental Deficiency*, vol. 87, (1982), pp.9–13.
30. Warren, S. F., Mulcahey, M. A., *Life planning for handicapped adults in Tennessee: Research findings and recommendations* (John F. Kennedy Center for Research on Education and Human Development, Peabody College, Vanderbilt University, Nashville, Tennessee, 1984).
31. Wertheimer, A., 'Living for the present: Older parents with a mentally handicapped person living at home', *Campaign for people with mental handicap* (CMH), Enquiry paper no. 9. (1981).
32. Wolfensberger, W., 'An overview of social role valorisation and some reflections on elderly mentally retarded persons' in Janicki, M. P., Wisniewski, H. M., (eds.), *Ageing and developmental disabilities: Issues and trends* (Paul Brookes, Baltimore, 1985).

This chapter was written on the basis of a grant from the Joseph Rowntree Memorial Trust to undertake an extensive review of the field of ageing and mental handicap which will appear as J. Hogg, S. Moss and D. Cooke (1988) *Ageing and Mental Handicap*, Chapman & Hall, London. The basis of the chapter is a paper given to the Groupe Belge D'Etude de L'Arrieration Mentale in June 1987.

PART FOUR

Total support as the basis for success

CHAPTER 14

Using generic and specialist medical services

Dr Yvonne Wiley
Senior Lecturer, Department of Mental Health,
University of Bristol

People with a mental handicap, like everyone else, need medical services; but because mental handicap is frequently associated with other medical conditions, they are likely throughout life to have a greater need for those services than the non-handicapped population. It is generally accepted that the generic services should be available and used if appropriate and in practice this is what happens. However, people with a mental handicap have the right to receive the best possible medical care and because this requires access to a wide range of specialist services, including those dealing exclusively with people with a mental handicap, then these must be available in every health district.

Generic medical services for children

Until a few years ago there was virtually no teaching about mental handicap in any medical school curriculum. Apart from areas touched on during the paediatric course, a doctor's entire teaching tended to consist of one visit to a large hospital where a few 'interesting syndromes' (sic!) were pointed out – an approach so likely to be counter-productive that it is amazing that any doctors chose to work in this field after qualifying. Happily, some did and all medical schools now include some relevant teaching about mental handicap. A number have established lecturers in mental handicap within their mental health departments and, at the time of writing, there are five chairs in the subject, with the hope of more being created before long. Paediatricians, too, have a greater awareness of the social and emotional impact of having a handicapped child.

This means that all doctors who qualify now have some knowledge of the causes of mental handicap, its associated conditions and their presentation and arguably, most important of all, an understanding of the needs of families who have a mentally handicapped member. For this reason general practitioners of the future are likely to feel more confident in providing the primary health care and are also more likely to be aware of how the specialised medical services can help and so make appropriate referrals. However, one has to remember that a general practitioner with 2,000 patients on his list is likely to have only about seven who have a mental handicap (unless he happens to have a number of group homes, hostels etc. in his area) registered with him and therefore is unable to develop a high level of expertise even if particularly interested: hence the reason for the back-up of specialist services for mentally handicapped people.

The first contact a person with a mental handicap has with the medical profession is at birth. Sometimes, but happily not very frequently, the handicap is caused by birth itself – either through intracranial haemorrhage, which is more likely to result from an unduly precipitate delivery or because the infant has suffered from anoxia, which can happen for a variety of reasons. Sometimes the baby suffers from an instantly recognisable syndrome, such as Down's Syndrome (and even in this case a diagnosis may not be possible without a chromosomal analysis). Even if the diagnosis seems obvious, the chromosomal analysis should be done as it will give information which will be used by the doctor for the purpose of genetic counselling. (There are a few types of chromosomal abnormality causing Down's Syndrome in which there is an increased likelihood of subsequent children being affected.) If there is no obvious abnormality in appearance the parents will not know immediately that their child is handicapped. Indeed, if it is a young mother's first baby, so that she had no idea what to expect as normal development, she may not suspect that anything is wrong for quite a long time after it would be obvious to professionals.

This illustrates the importance of regular attendance at baby clinics, run either at local authority centres or by the family's general practitioner, where development is monitored and a problem can be detected quickly. On the other hand, an experienced mother may well suspect that all is not well with her baby before the professionals can find any objective evidence of developmental delay – this is particularly so in autism, and professionals should always guard against thinking they know better than parents. Humility and willingness to listen are essential if mistakes are to be avoided! If a baby is not brought regularly to a clinic for routine checks, the general practitioner is likely to see the infant anyway for immunisation and will take the opportunity to assess the developmental level. Unfortunately because of the much publicised association between whooping cough vaccine and mental handicap some parents avoid all immunisations for their children. This is a great pity because the other immunisations are perfectly safe and can prevent tragic illnessess later as well as provide the opportunity for the doctor to complete a general examination of the baby.

The presenting symptoms in some cases of mental handicap may be that the baby has a fit. While this can be an alarming and distressing experience for a parent it should be remembered that the vast majority of fits in infancy are associated with minor illnesses which cause a raised temperature – a febrile convulsion – and have no significance for the future well-being of the child. Nevertheless, no fit in infancy should be treated lightly, and because all general practitioners see many children with febrile convulsions they will refer to a paediatrician those in whom they suspect that a more significant disorder underlies the fit.

Specialist medical services for children

These services are delivered in slightly different ways in various parts of the country. However, in every case once a child is suspected to suffer from a mental handicap it will be seen by a paediatrician for a full assessment. Some conditions are known to be associated with particular problems, such as abnormalities of skeletal development, muscular weakness, heart defects or impairment of hearing and/or vision. The paediatrician will in any case look for these associated handicaps and will if necessary liaise with colleagues who are specialists in these other fields of medicine. If a child has a mental handicap it is particularly important that any other handicaps (such as sight or hearing) are dealt with energetically so that they do not contribute further to the overall deficit. Indeed, an associated undiagnosed sensory impairment can mean that a child seems to be more severely mentally handicapped than he really is.

It may also be necessary for a surgeon to be involved – most commonly an orthopaedic or plastic surgeon – to correct associated physical abnormalities. A balance has to be struck between correcting a deformity and the pain and suffering such a procedure may cause; but in the main, corrective surgery is important, to lessen the handicaps borne by the child if at all possible.

The attitude of doctors at the time a diagnosis of mental handicap is made to parents is crucial. There is evidence that when people are given bad news of any sort they do not register anything that is said to them after the first few words. This may explain why some parents' recollection is that 'the doctor just told me the baby wasn't normal'. It may be that in a few appalling cases this was true, but it is more likely that the parents heard only those words and in their shock and distress missed everything else.

It is therefore essential that parents are seen together, and that interviews are repeated, so that they can be given as much information as possible and so that they have the opportunity to ask questions. They should be encouraged to make lists of things they want to ask about, as all too often when they are face to face with the professional concerned they forget much of what they wanted to say. The health visitor or community mental handicap nurse can be a key person in this. They visit the family at home and, in a more relaxed setting than clinic or doctor's surgery, can deal with questions and problems that arise. Community mental handicap nurses have a particular role here because of their knowledge of the wide range of mental handicap across all age groups and their personal practical experience of providing day-to-day care during their training.

It is worth noting that many of the questions parents ask relate not just to childhood but to the long-term outlook for their child and even the ultimate 'What will happen when I've gone?'. The sooner one tries to give a prognosis the less accurate it will be, but parents have the need, and the right, to have their questions fully answered and it is the author's experience that they prefer an honest 'I don't know' from the professional concerned to being fobbed off with half-truths or guesses.

All paediatricians, as described above, see children with a mental handicap and some centres have neuropaediatricians who are particularly skilled in assessing children with developmental delays and associated neurological deficits or conditions such as epilepsy. In some health districts children with a mental handicap may also be seen by the specialist psychiatrist in the psychiatry of mental handicap. These doctors have a particular contribution to make in the case of children who have associated problems in behaviour and can also help families with the emotional stress which is frequently, if not always, associated with having a mentally handicapped child. This experience can be seen as a form of bereavement and while many families adjust quickly others, although they love their handicapped child dearly, have greater difficulty in resolving the conflicting emotions and distress which they feel. This can involve non-handicapped brothers and sisters as well as parents and grandparents.

Psychiatrists who have trained in this field have been taught about the whole range of mental handicap, its causes and associated emotional, developmental and physical complexities as well as the genetic implications, if any. While working with the emotional aspects they are also, therefore, able to answer many of the other questions which may be raised by parents.

Adolescence can present particular difficulties in young people with a mental handicap. A number of factors make it problematic. Parents may find it hard to cope with the developing sexual awareness of someone whom they have until now perceived as a child, and may indeed deny its existence. Young people with mental handicaps become increasingly conscious of the differences between themselves and their siblings, whom they see going out with boy-friends or girl-friends and eventually getting married and having children. They may also resent their lack of independence from their parents. All these elements can contribute to considerable emotional turmoil at a time when, if the paediatrician has been the main medical support, the adolescent mentally handicapped person and his family may be without help when it is most needed. The value of involvement of the specialist medical service should not be forgotten.

Generic medical services for adults

Throughout life people with a mental handicap should have some form of regular medical checks. Those with more severe handicap may not complain of symptoms spontaneously. People who suffer from Down's Syndrome are particularly susceptible to some other medical conditions, notably chest infections. It is important that such infections are treated thoroughly in order to avoid the development of chronic infection in the lungs, known as bronchiectasis, which is a most distressing condition eventually leading to severe ill-health and death. Other medical conditions which occur more frequently in association with Down's Syndrome are diabetes and thyroid deficiency, both of which can be detected by routine examinations, and the necessary treatment initiated. People with Down's Syndrome also tend to develop obesity in adult life and apart from the obvious adverse effect this has on appearance, it has significance for general health and well-being and can encourage the development of associated medical problems such as hiatus hernia. It should therefore be countered by sensible dietary measures. One sometimes hears parents say they are reluctant to deprive their mentally handicapped child of what they see as their 'only' pleasure, in the form of sweets, cakes and desserts. Treats do not have to be cut out completely, but they should be kept for special occasions.

Some profoundly mentally handicapped people have multiple associated physical handicaps and consequent poor mobility and/or spasticity. They have particular need for skilled physiotherapy, which will be referred to in more detail under that heading.

Epilepsy is present in about 30% of people with severe mental handicap. However, control of fits is easier now than it used to be, and the medication used is less likely to have adverse side effects. Nevertheless, there are a few people in whom it is still very difficult or impossible to obtain adequate control, and even when fits can be reduced to a minimum, regular medical supervision and monitoring of the blood levels of the drugs used is essential. When blood levels become too high this can lead paradoxically to an increase in fits and without medical supervision parents or carers may mistakenly assume that drug levels are inadequate and increase the dose, leading to the development of toxic levels of the drug. Changes in dose of anticonvulsants should never be made without medical advice.

If a person with a mental handicap requires admission to a general hospital for investigation or treatment, perhaps surgical, it is helpful if a relative or familiar carer can stay with them, particularly at the beginning and at times of stress such as during the immediate post-operative period. Apart from the reassurance this affords it can help staff who may have no experience in mental handicap to communicate more easily and appropriately.

Specialist medical services for adults

The need for good medical care throughout life has already been outlined. However, people with a mental handicap may, like others, suffer from superimposed psychiatric illness and are more likely than non-handicapped people to have a range of emotional disorders or to present with difficulties in behaviour (currently called challenging behaviours because they present a challenge to the skills of carers and professionals alike).

The psychiatrist specialising in the psychiatry of mental handicap has been trained to diagnose and treat emotional and psychiatric problems and should be consulted if and when they arise. Some parts of the country are still under-provided with these specialist psychiatrists and in this case patients may be referred to a general psychiatrist. However, even well-known psychiatric illnesses tend to have an unusual presentation in people who are mentally handicapped and may give particular difficulties in diagnosis. For that reason the specialist psychiatrist has a valuable contribution to make. He may see patients referred (by GP, social worker or other professional) in a variety of settings, depending on local circumstances, and will certainly want to discuss matters with other family members or carers. If epilepsy first presents in adult life that, too, can be referred to the specialist service although it may be referred to a neurologist who works predominantly with people who do not have a mental handicap.

Whatever the condition, it can often be dealt with as an outpatient. If medication is prescribed the doctor will ensure that it is in a form which is most acceptable to the individual (e.g. syrup may be preferable to tablets). Mildly mentally handicapped people can sometimes be given responsibility for taking their own medication, and tablets can be issued in a container which is sectioned in the days of the week so that mistakes are minimised. In the case of some medication prescribed for psychiatric conditions, and always in the case of epilepsy, it will be necessary to have tests to monitor the blood levels. The importance of this will be explained to parents or carers, along with a description of possible side effects so that they can be looked for, since the person with a mental handicap may not spontaneously complain of such symptoms. In some cases side effects may be unavoidable, but are often outweighed by the benefits of the medication.

Occasionally it is not possible to treat the psychiatric condition or epilepsy adequately as an out-patient and admission to hospital becomes necessary. This may be in a general psychiatric unit or in a mental handicap hospital, most of which retain either beds or units to provide assessment and psychiatric treatment on a short or medium-term basis. Most health districts accept that there will continue to be a need for this specialised facility, although in future it may in some districts be sited in a general psychiatric hospital.

Admission to hospital has the advantage of continuous nursing and medical supervision and the possibility of monitoring and changing drug regimes to achieve the best possible result for the individual. If the patient refuses to accept admission it is very occasionally necessary, and in their best interests, to admit compulsorily under a section of the Mental Health Act and in this case their rights are protected under the law as applies to anyone for whom compulsory admission to hospital becomes necessary.

Dental treatment

Good dental hygiene and care of the teeth are if anything more important in people with a mental handicap than in the rest of the population. They have an increased incidence of dental malformation and, because of the possible difficulty in persuading them to tolerate the essentially uncomfortable procedures involved in conservation dentistry (e.g. fillings), it is sensible to avoid the development of caries in the first place. If the family dentist does not feel able, for whatever reason, to provide routine dental care, then it can be provided either by a dental hospital or the community dental service. There are also in many parts of the country specialist dental departments which have a long-established association with the mental handicap hospitals and these provide an excellent, experienced and sympathetic service for people with a mental handicap.

Other professionals in the medical services

The 'professions allied to medicine' (psychologists, nurses, occupational therapists, physiotherapists and speech therapists) have a substantial role to play in a comprehensive medical service for people with a mental handicap, and work with all ages and all levels of ability and disability. There are areas of overlap in their work but each profession has a special and unique contribution. Community Mental Handicap Teams are being developed throughout the country and the professions allied to medicine work within these teams. The roles of the various professionals are outlined in the following paragraphs.

Clinical psychologists

After completing a degree in psychology, clinical psychologists undergo further training in the application of psychology in psychiatry including the psychiatry of mental handicap. They are usually based in a hospital but increasingly work as members of a Community Mental Handicap Team. The assessments which they make include formal psychometric testing (IQ tests) but more commonly today cover a very wide range of tests for intellectual ability, personality, and social functioning. Many clinical psychologists have had training in computer technology and take a key role in setting up and maintaining registers. However the role of the psychologist is by no means limited to testing clients. They have an invaluable contribution to make in planning and advising on various treatment programmes, usually based on behaviour modification techniques. They also frequently work, either alone or with a psychiatrist, with families who may have emotional problems in coping with their mentally handicapped child, and advise families on approaches to the management of behaviour problems such as sleeping or eating disorders.

Community nurses

The mental handicap nurse working in the community contributes to the service in many and varied ways. It should not be forgotten that these nurses are able to offer nursing skills in the general sense as well as having particular knowledge of mental handicap. They undertake nursing treatments such as giving injections or enemas, and in so doing may relate to a hospital consultant or directly to the family doctor. They monitor medication and keep records of conditions such as epilepsy or diabetes, alerting the doctor when further medical attention is required.

Community mental handicap nurses perform a valuable liaison role between the various services which may be involved in the life of a person with mental handicap: school, hospital and family doctor. However, as well as these general nursing duties, the mental handicap nurse frequently undertakes other therapeutic interventions. Many are trained in the Portage scheme and all have experience in carrying out and advising families on behaviour modification programmes planned by the clinical psychologist or psychiatrist. Perhaps most important of all, the community mental handicap nurse, with such a wide range of knowledge in the field, becomes a trusted friend and support to families who have a mentally handicapped member – a contribution which is difficult to measure but is none the less real and valuable.

Occupational therapists

During their training all occupational therapists do some work in psychiatric settings and many have the opportunity to work in the field of mental handicap. They all have training in mental handicap which equips them to identify and treat specific neurological and developmental deficits which may accompany the handicap. Their skills and techniques also improve the social functioning of clients. Their contribution to the Community Mental Handicap Team is to carry out detailed assessments of a person's abilities and to plan and implement programmes to encourage development of skills in a systematic way, in line with the normal developmental stages.

Occupational therapists also advise on the provision of appropriate aids and appliances, frequently tailored to individual needs. Although occupational therapy departments also provide a wide range of occupational and social activities, occupational therapists have moved a long way from the old image (which was never quite accurate in any case) of basket-making and knitting instructors. They have a considerable therapeutic input and their skills are essential in preparing hospital patients to move into the community and in setting up and equipping houses for people who may have multiple handicaps.

Physiotherapists

Mental handicap is sometimes associated with physical handicaps. These may be the result of associated physical abnormalities of development, such as skeletal or bony deformities, or may be secondary to impaired functioning of the central nervous system, as with spasticity, hypotonicity and abnormal involuntary movements of muscles. For all these handicaps skilled physiotherapy is required, either to improve function or to minimise deterioration.

Physiotherapists also work closely with orthopaedic surgeons. This is sometimes at the time of surgical intervention but is most frequently a long-term involvement in the provision of appliances such as remedial footwear or mobility aids (walking frames, wheelchairs etc.). Physiotherapists work with patients both in individual treatment regimes, with or without specialised equipment, and in group activities. In the case of very profoundly handicapped patients who are particularly prone to chest infections it is sometimes necessary to have daily physiotherapy to keep the lungs clear and the physiotherapist is usually happy to advise carers on the most beneficial techniques to use, when it is not possible for the physiotherapist to give the treatment personally.

Speech therapists

These should perhaps be more accurately known as communication therapists! While their skills are most commonly thought of as helping people to speak more clearly they have a much wider role. Because their training helps them to understand the functioning of mouth and throat muscles as well as equipping them to identify a variety of hearing impairments which may be present, they contribute to the well-being of those people with a mental handicap who, because of developmental deficits, will never learn to speak.

One aspect of this input which may not readily spring to mind is the help speech therapists give in educating profoundly handicapped people to chew and swallow. Because there are not enough speech therapists to meet the demand they frequently work with parents or other carers to educate them in useful feeding techniques.

They also undertake detailed assessments analysing the reasons why speech may be impaired, reasons which may range from defects in hearing to very specific muscular and neurological abnormalities in the speech-producing organs. Treatment regimes are then planned based on these assessments.

Speech therapists also work on programmes of non-verbal communications such as MAKATON sign-language and the reduction in frustration when someone is able to communicate in this way is one of the most rewarding aspects of their work.

CHAPTER 15

Designing environments

Mary Dalgleish, PhD
*Independent Research Worker, Department of Psychiatry,
University of Sheffield*

The environment in which people live and work has been shown to have a powerful influence on behaviour (Canter and Canter, 1979). This chapter briefly considers current guidance on the design of appropriate residential and day-care environments for mentally handicapped adults in relation to evaluation studies of design features.

Residential environments

Current design guidance

The Government's commitment to the transfer of mentally handicapped people to community care was stressed in the 'Care in the Community' Green Paper (DHSS, 1981). 'Care in the Community' was defined as meaning an integrated service network to support mentally handicapped people according to their individual needs in a setting – own home, sharing someone else's home, group home, etc. – which provides the maximum opportunities for ordinary living among ordinary people. Housing agencies, local authority social services departments, health authorities, voluntary bodies and private individuals were all seen to have roles in providing such accommodation.

Health authorities have a much reduced role in providing residential care than that envisaged in 1971 in the Government White Paper 'Better Services for the Mentally Handicapped' (DHSS, 1971). The 1980 review (DHSS, 1980a) concluded that few districts were likely to need more than 150 health care places. In 1985 it was stated that health authorities should aim to accommodate eventually in small, homely units based in local communities all mentally handicapped people requiring care in a health setting, except possibly some with special needs (DHSS, 1985).

Current guidance thus emphasises that there should be nothing 'special' about the residential environments created for the majority of mentally handicapped people. This may seem surprising given

that mentally handicapped people often do have particular difficulties in everyday life, difficulties which perhaps could be
overcome more easily within a specially-designed, therapeutic
environment.

Designing special residential environments

Mentally handicapped people can be regarded as needing help in
learning the basic tasks of living, and practice in these tasks in a
realistic setting might be seen as appropriate 'therapy'. For example,
a situation wherein individuals have to share a 30-bed dormitory,
have communal washing and bathing facilities, and clothing from a
central store, is clearly less homely and provides fewer opportunities
for personal choice and decision-making than one where people
have their own room, have privacy when washing and bathing and
have facilities to keep, wear and care for their own clothes and
personal possessions. Further, while energetic care staff may be
able to provide stimulating conditions in even the most sterile
environment, this would seem more likely to occur in favourable
physical settings. For example, a considerable amount of effort
would be required to undertake domestic training programmes in a
building where the kitchen has catering-style equipment geared to
providing large numbers of meals a day.

Before 1971, the majority of mentally handicapped people
requiring residential care were placed in hospital. By 1971 it had
become clear that there were considerable problems in some long
stay mental handicap hostels (e.g. Ely) and that the physical environment was important in adding to or detracting from a home-
like atmosphere. 'Better Services' (DHSS, 1971) proposed a radical
shift in emphasis away from institutional hospital care to care
'within the community'. Three specific groups were identified,
each believed to have particular residential requirements. Some
people, those with the most severe handicaps, additional physical
handicaps or severe behaviour problems, were believed still to
require hospital care but this was to be provided in smaller units
associated with general hospitals, rather than specialist hospitals,
and in units promoting a homelike, domestic environment. Other
people, with less severe handicaps (less obvious physical handicaps,
possibly some degree of incontinence and behaviour problems)
were believed to require limited medical and nursing supervision. It
was thought that this could best be provided in small, community-
based health service units. Those remaining, who could be cared
for within a normal home if such a home were available to them,
were believed to be most appropriately placed in local authority
social services hostels or group homes.

The Sheffield Development Project provided a large-scale testing-
ground for some of the principles of the White Paper and a major

feature of the project was the design and provision of new purpose-built buildings appropriate to the three groups identified: hospital units for the most severely handicapped; community-based health service hostels for those requiring limited medical and nursing supervision; local authority hostels for those who could be cared for within a normal home if such were available. Comprehensive design guidance was developed for each of the three types of building. Although all were larger than would now be rec-ommended, at the time the scale of accommodation was a sub-stantial reduction on existing provision. It was suggested that the smaller hospital units should be under 200 beds, sub-grouped into 24s and further divided into groups of 12 for adults (eight for children); the hostels were generally for a total of 24, and in the case of the health service hostels, further subdivided into three eight-person houses. Buildings based on this guidance sprang up in other parts of the country such as Peterborough, Rotherham, Dudley and Enfield.

Results of evaluation studies

Research was carried out to assess the success of these new special buildings and their role in encouraging community care. The variety of units provided under the Sheffield project, along with the unit at Peterborough, allowed an evaluation of features of design, planning and organisation (DHSS Works Group 1981a, 1980a).

The residential needs of the three 'types' of client identified appeared to be similar, despite the different environments provided. For all, smaller sub-groupings of four to six residents were preferred by staff. Staff believed that these groups should be completely separate, preferably in their own, self-contained house, but at least, and most important, with their own domestic-style kitchen and dining area. In such situations, the skills which had been practised in carefully-constructed domestic training situations became the reality of day-to-day life. As well as contributing to a more homelike environment, the provision of completely separate houses for small groups affords greater flexibility in that as needs change, single houses can be taken over by different users.

If care is really to be 'in the community', the use of community amenities must be feasible. The studies in Sheffield highlighted the importance of residential units being in a position from which community facilities might be easily accessible in order to encourage their use by residents. This includes avoiding major traffic hazards. One unit in Sheffield was virtually cut off from the surrounding community by a fast dual-carriageway. Accessibility and traffic hazards should be important considerations in the allocation of accommodation within the community. Accessibility can be assessed by calculating the distance from the unit of various com-

munity amenities such as the post office, park, shops, day centre
and bus stops (DHSS Works Group, 1981a).

A disadvantage of purpose-built residential units can be the
physical clash with surrounding housing: local residents' unfavour-
able views about new provision appeared to relate more to its
appearance than to its mentally handicapped occupants. Further,
when buildings had unusual features such as a different type of
brickwork or shape of window, some neighbours rationalised that
the mentally handicapped occupants must 'need' such special accommodation. The different bricks were seen as perhaps being
especially strong and the windows shaped in that way to prevent
residents falling out. In other words, the destigmatising potential of
being sited in the community was lost. The hostel which prompted
the most favourable comments from the neighbours was one which
looked like three ordinary houses and had been built at the same
time as (and in similar materials to) the surrounding estate (DHSS
Works Group, 1979). But, even when the component houses of a
hostel look like the surrounding ordinary housing, their positioning within one site can mark them out as different: one hostel had
its three eight-bed houses and two staff houses all positioned within
one boundary wall, served by a single main gateway bearing the
name of the hostel. A simple rearrangement, giving each
house access from the road, might have altered the institutional
character.

Thus, research indicated that what many staff users of these
special buildings wanted was ordinary housing sited within the
community. Many schemes have successfully utilised ordinary
housing (Shearer, 1981; DHSS Works Group, 1981b). It does
appear that, *given appropriate staff support*, the majority of mentally
handicapped people – perhaps all – could be accommodated in
ordinary housing. Policy guidance points to, and the trend is
towards, this sort of provision rather than larger and more traditional settings (DHSS, 1985, p.14).

An example of how an institutional feeling can be created in even
ordinary housing is the fire precaution debate. There are numerous
ways in which rigidly applied fire regulations can affect the type of
environment created: residents not being allowed duvets; highly
obtrusive fire extinguishers and signs being installed; additional
firedoors added; external fire-escapes marking the house out from
its neighbours. There is increasing realisation that the need for fire
precautions in residential care homes must be weighed carefully
against the need to maintain a homely and non-institutional atmosphere (DHSS, 1985, p.7). The issue comes down to a general one
concerning the increased risks of ordinary living versus the
highly protected environment previously considered appropriate.
Ordinary housing, with, for example, accessible kitchen equip-

ment and sited close to roads, contains greater potential risks than hospitals or many hostels. With sufficient and appropriate staff supervision it is these 'risks' which can provide the challenging situations necessary to stimulate the development of skills.

Special groups

There are a small number of mentally handicapped people who may require special provision due to additional physical handicaps or severe behaviour problems. Some mentally handicapped people with physical handicaps may require special facilities created by adapting ordinary housing, just as many non-mentally handicapped people do. To be responsive to the needs of the users of a service such specialised facilities should be planned around the current needs of each individual. A local case register might indicate the number of people having a particular problem (for instance, being non-ambulant) and the potential numbers requiring residential care might be estimated, but exactly when a particular individual will require the care, and where he or she would like it, and the exact nature of the special aids required, make it impossible to plan ahead in this way. There are examples of special facilities and equipment incorporated into units in line with an expected need in the population, but never used by the eventual residents. Far better to adapt a property as and when required. Even the necessity for purpose-built accommodation does not preclude integration with ordinary housing: such accommodation has been successfully incorporated within a new (ordinary) housing scheme for individuals with physical handicaps (Davis, 1981).

For the very small number of people with severe behavioural problems, the official position appears to be that there may be a case for specially designed provision. The Sheffield studies found that such residents tended to be grouped together and lived in units with less domestic environments *even where physically similar accommodation had originally been provided for all residents*. This was often due to wear and tear on fittings, indicating the difficulty in maintaining an ordinary domestic environment under such pressure. While some would argue that given sufficient and appropriate staff support, no special physical facilities would be required, others might opt for providing a small unit on a regional or supraregional basis. Another possibility is the provision of specialised units for intensive therapy for a limited time. Such issues, including examples of therapeutic situations, have been considered in the DHSS report, 'Helping Mentally Handicapped People with Special Problems' (1984).

Thus, despite a possible need for special residential provision for a very small number of clients, for the large majority appropriate staff support within ordinary housing appears to be considered the most suitable environment. The adequacy of staffing and of staff support systems is of paramount importance given the potential isolation of these smaller housing units. There is a strong case for seeing residential provision as becoming the domain of the local authority and housing agencies, and for discouraging health and local authorities from building purpose-built accommodation. Where it is felt that a community unit-type building is necessary, perhaps for special groups or as a respite care/resource centre, guidance is available (DHSS, 1980b; DHSS Works Group, 1982). This encourages many of the domestic aspects raised above, including a preference for individually-sited sub-units. However, there seems to be no reason why this type of facility could not be provided/funded by housing agencies/associations on behalf of health authorities or social services departments.

Day care environments

Current design guidance

Guidance on day care facilities has lagged behind that on residential facilities although any move to ordinary housing in the wider community relies heavily on a corresponding increase in day services. There are those who claim that the old mental handicap hospitals greatly benefited the more severely mentally handicapped people because of the sheltered community created with day facilities on site. (There are examples of private schemes such as Home Farm Trust and Ravenswood where total communities have been developed, often based on agricultural and craft industries.) The concern is that unless sufficient and appropriate day facilities are provided, some people could be moved out of hospitals into the wider community and end up being isolated and deprived of appropriate experiences during the day. Lack of day care facilities is also one of the factors which can eventually drive families to seek full-time care for a mentally handicapped member.

Although there is valuable information available about provision for special care/special needs for the most severely handicapped clients who have traditionally attended hospital day care centres (DHSS, 1984), there is no official design guidance. Consequently, there has been a range of differing solutions with varying space standards. New local authority special care units are frequently planned as an extension to an existing adult training centre (ATC) or as an annexe to a new one rather than as a fully-integrated part of a centre. This may be because the only official design guidance for ATCs (DHSS, 1972) recommends that ATCs be designed, equipped and organised on workshop lines with smaller areas to provide for domestic training and education. This situation does not appear to lend itself easily to the task of including people with special needs in the ATC/SEC system. This official design guidance, however, is in conflict with the National Development Group's (1977) recommendation that a centre should fulfil many functions in addition to work training, including a 'special care section'.

More recently planned centres are providing specialist resource areas. The range of facilities and services offered to *all* clients can thus be extended by making particular provision for people with severe physical or sensory handicaps and people with severe behaviour problems. Equally, people with special needs can be encouraged to experience the use of other facilities of the centre. Such centres can be geared around a more flexible approach to the provision of day facilities for mentally handicapped people within the community. They represent a distinct shift from the notion of a traditional ATC, providing an 'open' system of opportunities linked to existing resources in the community such as FE colleges, adult education centres, community recreational and cultural facilities, work experience groups and voluntary clubs and societies.

Designing for special needs

Day provision for this group should be designed to incorporate learning situations and educational challenges which, when used with individual training programmes, can assist better functioning and reduced dependency. The environment must therefore support and enhance progress. Two hospital day-care environments were created in Sheffield as part of the development project. One consisted of inter-linked open-plan spaces while the other had a range of self-contained areas. Research carried out in these and other day centres for profoundly and severely handicapped adults raised a number of issues relevant in the design of specialist resource areas (DHSS Works Group, 1980b).

Staff tended to work with groups of six to eight clients (fewer than anticipated when the buildings were designed). Staff felt strongly that small groupings were essential if anything of therapeutic value were to be achieved. Their views were supported by observational studies which showed that the more clients present in one space, the fewer were 'engaged' (busy, involved). The observational studies also indicated that levels of client engagement and the amount of communication that clients received from staff were related to design features, being lower in larger, more open areas, and in areas with an integral circulation route. The levels were lower when two groups were organised simultaneously in a large open area than when the same groups each had their own self-contained room.

The clear indication is that self-contained spaces suitable for small groups are more effective than larger, more open areas. Regarding appropriate size: complaints were made at one centre that the rooms, measuring 28 square metres, were too small; at another with rooms measuring 42 square metres, no complaints were recorded. Regarding shape: staff criticised irregular-shaped areas with features which allowed clients to be out of sight of staff, and experimentation with a partition has demonstrated (Sandhu *et al.*, 1976) that a more or less square room is more favourable to staff contact than an elongated one.

Research has also highlighted the importance of providing areas for one-to-one work. These should be *separate* from the main activity spaces. Bays adjoining a room used concurrently by other clients could not be used for this purpose due to difficulty in maintaining clients' concentration and attention in the midst of distracting stimuli.

The above considerations may suggest a rather uninteresting environment with several smallish, squarish group rooms, some smaller one-to-one rooms, and avoidance of through-routes in activity spaces, suggested to provide 'bewildering and meaningless' movement for the severely mentally handicapped clients (*ibid.*). Indeed, it has in the past been suggested that mentally handicapped people would be helped by an environment as non-stimulating as possible, without pictures, flowers and other distractions, and that enrichment of the environment might lead to bewilderment. However, a number of studies have shown (e.g. Levy and McLeod, 1977) that an enriched and stimulating physical environment has measurable benefits to the client. Suggestions about how such environmental enrichment might be achieved in special care units for children include: 'greater use of colour and texture on walls, ceilings and floors to help children with perceptual difficulties; greater variety between and within rooms to encourage exploration and movement; and opportunities for social involvement and withdrawal, for experiment and surprises' (Sandhu *et al.*, 1976).

The day centres were carefully designed to allow flexibility and versatility of the use of spaces. However, areas were taken over for specific functions – such as woodwork or physiotherapy –and were often not seen to be available to other groups even when empty, generally due to the specialised equipment present. Fixed or large equipment thus appears to reduce the potential flexibility of spaces. A frequently raised concern was about the safety of physically frail clients when sharing facilities with the more active clients. Both groups place considerable demands on space.

The broad aims in planning for this group should thus be for sufficient self-contained spaces and for spaces that can be used flexibly for a number of different functions. Consideration must therefore be given to the following:

1. Provision of spaces of a suitable size for small group or individual work.

2. Areas of a shape that can be easily supervised.
3. The avoidance of fixed equipment.
4. Minimising noises from and views into adjoining areas.
5. Providing versatility of use.
6. Provision of sufficient area to allow the separation of the physically handicapped from more active clients, to allow space for prone clients or for wheelchair users, for mobility training and for storage.
7. Provision of easy access to external recreation space.

The plan (see Fig. 15.1) provides a suggested arrangement for a 15-place resource area suitable for clients with special needs and incorporating many of the above considerations. Most authorities are now coming to plan resource areas within a range of 10, 15, or 20 places.

The following quotation is reproduced from 'Helping handicapped people with special problems', DHSS, 1984.

'Activities can be planned to take place in one large multipurpose area but it is preferable to use smaller linked and related spaces. This makes it easier to organise clients in sub-groups as well as carry out activities with individual clients. Furthermore, linked and related spaces, if designed to provide flexibility of shape and to allow versatility of use should encourage staff to combine spaces for activities involving the whole group or to use a range of self-contained rooms for small group or one-to-one activities, whilst being able to supervise other spaces. The small rooms could also be used by specialist visitors (e.g. speech therapists) on a sessional basis although this would mean that the various disciplines would have to work flexibly in multi-purpose spaces. There are two particular advantages to this kind of arrangement: it aids communication between professionals working in the centre and it avoids the provision of potentially underused specialist rooms.

'The sub-division of space is usually discussed in relation to the need to separate out people with particular handicapping conditions; in particular the protection of the more frail, physically handicapped clients from those who are very active and robust. However, there are advantages in bringing the various sub-groups together for some activities. Space should therefore be arranged such that both sub-division and total integration is possible.

'The plan illustrates how spaces can be planned so that they may be used in a variety of ways. Many other planning arrangements are possible – or even preferable – but this plan does provide environments which are not only fun to be in but which have potential for staff and clients to exploit them to the full. It is

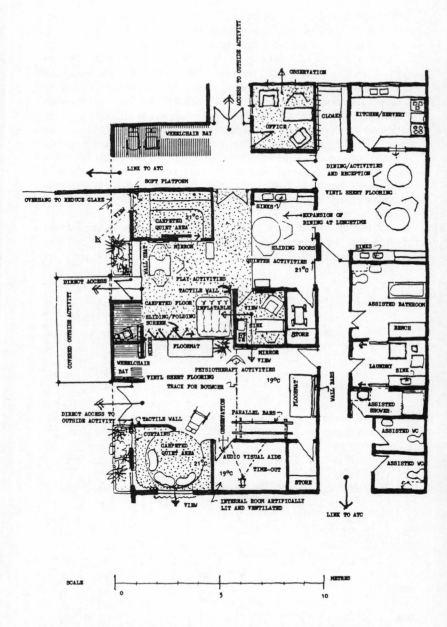

Fig. 15.1 A suggestion for a layout for a resource area providing 15 places. (Reproduced from 'Helping handicapped people with special problems', DHSS, 1984.)

intended that the use of spaces shown on the plans will be decided in advance but they should also be flexible enough for individual improvisations.

'A unit for a high dependency group with mixed disabilities within the broad category of severely mentally handicapped people poses particular problems. Design features which have advantages for some clients are hazardous for others. For example, full-height glazed panels in walls or partitions designed to allow supervision or to allow people with hearing loss to have more visual clues may be dangerous to someone who is partially sighted; or a room planned with hard wall and floor surfaces for hard play activities may produce a noisy environment in which people with impaired hearing will have difficulty in comprehending words and sounds.

'The plan allows a wide range of environments which take account of the disabilities likely to be present and which permit a wide range of programmes to meet clients' needs. The plan provides for variety in the layout of spaces and in how they are defined by a choice of materials, textures and decorations. Soft, carpeted areas are designed for quiet activities and small self-contained rooms for one-to-one sessions should be accoustically well insulated. This will provide a different sound environment for different activities. Different environments are not solely achieved by the provision of a variety of spaces. Consideration should also be given to different levels of illumination, variations in the amount of natural lighting and room temperatures. It must be borne in mind that each space is intended to present a specific ambience to be experienced when moving from one to another.'

Further reading

1. Canter, D., Canter, S., *Designing for therapeutic environments: a review of research* (Chichester, Wiley, 1979).
2. Davis, K., '28–38 Grove Road: accommodation and care in a community setting', in Brechin, A., Liddiard, P., Swain, J., *Handicap in a Social World* (Hodder and Stoughton, 1981).
3. DHSS, *Better services for the mentally handicapped,* (Cmnd 4683, HMSO, 1971).
4. DHSS, *Local Authority Building Note 5,* (1972).
5. DHSS, *Progress, problems and priorities: a review of mental handicap services since the 1971 white paper,* (1980a).
6. DHSS, *Health Service residential accommodation for the mentally handicapped,* (HN(80)21 Annex III, 1980b).
7. DHSS, *Care in the community: a consultative document on moving resources for care in England,* (1981).
8. DHSS, *Helping mentally handicapped people with special prob-*

lems: report of a DHSS study team, (A review of current approaches to meeting the needs of mentally handicapped people with special problems.) (DHSS, 1984).

9. DHSS, *Community care – with special reference to mentally ill and mentally handicapped people*, (Government response to the second report from the social services committee, 1984–85 session, Cmnd 9674, HMSO, 1985).

10. DHSS Works Group, *Mental health buildings evaluation reports on development projects for mentally handicapped people*, (obtainable from Room 517, Euston Tower, 286 Euston Road, London NW1 3DN).

11. DHSS Works Group, *Community reaction to local buildings*, (S3, 1979).

12. DHSS Works Group, *Childrens' and adults' units at the Gloucester Centre*, (P1, 1980a).

13. DHSS Works Group, *Hospital day care for adults*, (S6, 1980b).

14. DHSS Works Group, *Adult residential accommodation*, (S8, 1981a).

15. DHSS Works Group, *Pamphlet 1: Residential facilities for mentally handicapped children*, (1981b).

16. DHSS Works Group, *Pamphlet 2: Health services residential accommodation for severely mentally handicapped people: how to make the most of current design guidance*, (1982).

17. Levy, E., McLeod, W., 'The effects of environmental design on adolescents in an institution', *Mental Retardation*, vol. 15, (1977), pp.28–32.

18. National Development Group, *Pamphlet No. 5: Day services for mentally handicapped adults*, (1977).

19. Sandhu, J. S., Hendricks-Jansen, H., *Environmental design for handicapped children* (Saxon House, 1976).

20. Shearer, A., *Bringing mentally handicapped children out of hospital* (Kings' Fund Centre, Project Paper 30, 1981).

CHAPTER 16

State benefits and other financial help

James Ross
Formerly Director, Welfare and Counselling Service, MENCAP

People who are mentally handicapped are amongst the most vulnerable members of our society and few of them are able to understand which services and benefits they are entitled to or where to apply for them. Nobody has the statutory or legal responsibility to advise them. They depend upon other people such as parents, carers, professionals or friends to advise and help them. In this chapter we examine the main sources of financial help which people with a mental handicap may be able to claim.

State social security benefits

The majority of people who have a mental handicap are entitled to receive support from the state social security system. These benefits are non-contributory and are based on Acts of Parliament. Some are to help with living expenses and others are to help with the extra costs disability may cause (e.g. mobility allowance). Where do you begin?

First, find out where the local social security office is. The address can be found in the telephone directory under 'Health and Social Security, Department of'. Details of the various benefits and claim forms are available at social security offices, where help and advice may be sought. The DHSS publishes a wide range of leaflets about benefits and the rules that apply to them. Most leaflets are available at local social security offices or they will order them for you, or they can be ordered direct from the DHSS Leaflet Unit, PO Box 21, Stanmore, Middlesex, HA7 1AY.

The main benefits and how to claim them

Brief details are given below about the main benefits and how to claim them (see also Table 16.1). If you require further help ask at your local social security office or Citizens' Advice Bureau. If a claim is refused and you think this is unreasonable or unfair, you have the right to appeal to a Social Security Appeals Tribunal

Table 16.1 Easy reference chart to main benefits.

Benefit	Who is it for?	Who pays it?	How is it claimed?
Income Support	To help people who do not have enough money to live on. Intended to meet regular weekly needs.	Local DHSS office	By letter, postal claim forms or a form inside the leaflet SB1
Social Fund	To help with exceptional expenses which are difficult to pay from regular income.	Local DHSS office	On form SF300
Severe Disablement Allowance	Those without NI contributions to qualify for sickness and invalidity benefits.	Local DHSS office	Claim form inside leaflet
Attendance Allowance	Those needing a lot of care or supervision (for at least six months).	Attendance Allowance Unit, Norcross, Blackpool	Application form inside the AA leaflet
Mobility Allowance	Those with great walking difficulties or who cannot walk at all.	Mobility Allowance Unit, Norcross, Blackpool	The form is in the MA leaflet
Invalid Care Allowance	Those caring for someone who gets Attendance Allowance.	Invalid Care Allowance Unit, Norcross, Blackpool	The form is in the ICA leaflet

(SSAT) where the matter will be decided by an Adjudication Officer (AO). Remember, an appeal must be lodged within 28 days. Advice and help about appeals is available from most Citizens' Advice Bureaux or from MENCAP.

Attendance Allowance

Attendance Allowance is a cash allowance paid to people who are severely disabled, physically or mentally, and need plenty of attention or supervision from others. It is not means-tested and is tax-free. No National Insurance contributions are needed. It is paid to disabled people or to the parents of disabled children. People who receive the allowance can spend it as they choose.

ELIGIBILITY

Entitlement to Attendance Allowance depends on the attention or supervision disabled people need, not on the degree or cause of their disablement or on the actual help they receive. Two people might have exactly the same degree of disability, but one might qualify and the other not, because of the different extent to which they have been able to adapt to their disability. People may qualify for the allowance if they fulfil the following criteria:

1. **Age**: applicants must be over the age of two years. Children less than two years old cannot qualify. An adult (generally the mother) must claim on behalf of a child under 16 years. There are no upper age limits.
2. **Employment**: disabled people doing paid work may qualify.
3. **Residence**: the disabled person must be normally resident in Great Britain (England, Scotland and Wales).
4. **Accommodation**: applicants should not be living in hospital or in a home or school which is run or sponsored by an agency of local or central government. However, the allowance can be paid on a daily basis for periods spent away from hospital or residential accommodation (e.g. weekends spent at home, holidays and visits to relatives). The Attendance Allowance Unit should be told about such absences in advance so that payment can be considered. If there is to be a regular pattern of home leave, payments can be arranged accordingly. People living alone can claim.
5. **Disability**: applicants must be so severely disabled that for at least six months they have needed the following:
   (a) Frequent attention throughout the day in connection with their bodily functions (e.g. eating, washing, using the toilet), or continual supervision throughout the day in order to avoid substantial danger to themselves or others.
   (b) Prolonged or repeated attention during the night in con-

nection with their bodily functions, or continual supervision throughout the night in order to avoid substantial danger to themselves or others.

People who need attention or supervision both day and night get the higher rate of allowance. People who need attention or supervision by day or night get the lower rate of allowance.

Children under 16 years of age must need substantially more attention or supervision then a child of the same age normally requires.

CLAIMING

The claim form is attached to the Attendance Allowance leaflet available from social security offices. Applicants should post the completed form to the appropriate social security office.

A parent or guardian should claim for a child under 16 years of age. If both parents live with the disabled child the mother should make the claim, though both parents are entitled to cash the payments. If an adult disabled person cannot complete the form, another adult can do it for him, but the disabled person should sign the form if possible. The Secretary of State may appoint someone to act on behalf of disabled people who are unable to act for themselves because of their physical or mental incapacity. When this happens the person appointed is responsible for dealing with all the National Insurance affairs of the disabled person, including claiming and receiving benefit, and is also responsible for notifying changes in circumstances which affect benefit. Any benefit received under such an appointment must be used in the interests, and for the well-being, of the disabled person. Disabled people who are able to handle their own affairs but have difficulty in getting to the post office to cash their order book can arrange for other people to collect their money for them.

ASSOCIATED BENEFITS

Payment of Attendance Allowance is used by other schemes as a way of confirming disablement. People receiving Attendance Allowance may also qualify for the following:

1. British Rail card for disabled people.
2. Exemptions from vehicle excise duty (in some cases).
3. Supplementary Benefit heating additions.
4. Severe Disablement Allowance (if of working age and incapable of work).
5. Higher needs allowance in calculating entitlement to Housing Benefit.

Disabled people are exempted from road tax if they are unable or virtually unable to walk, and have a car registered in their name but are too disabled to drive. Special arrangements about registration apply for children. For further information, apply to your local DHSS office.

Invalid Care Allowance (ICA)

ICA is a cash allowance for people of working age who are unable to go to work because they are looking after a severely disabled person at home. It is therefore an allowance paid to carers, rather than directly to people with disabilities. The applicant does not have to be related to the disabled person or live at the same address and the allowance is not means tested. Although ICA is liable to income tax, no National Insurance contributions are needed, and while ICA is being paid the claimant is credited with contributions.

ELIGIBILITY

1. **Age**: applicants must be over 16 years of age and under pension age (65 years for a man, 60 years for a woman) when they claim. People who have qualified for ICA before they reach pension age can continue receiving all or some of the allowance after pension age if they do not qualify for a retirement pension of at least the rate of ICA.
2. **Residence**: applicants must normally live in the UK. They must also have been present in England, Scotland, Wales or Northern Ireland for at least 26 weeks during the previous 12 months.
3. **Care**: applicants must spend at least 25 hours each week caring for someone who is receiving one of the following:
   (a) Attendance Allowance (at the higher or lower rate).
   (b) Constant Attendance Allowance (at the normal maximum rate of above) associated with a war or services pension or an industrial disablement pension or an allowance under the Pneumoconiosis, Byssiniosis and Miscellaneous Diseases Benefit Scheme.

CLAIMING

Claimants should fill in the claim form at the back of the Invalid Care Allowance leaflet (N1.212) which can be obtained from their social security office. They should send the form to the ICA Unit in Blackpool. The address is: Department of Health and Social Security, Invalid Care Allowance Unit, North Fylde Central Office, Norcross, Blackpool, Lancashire, FY5 3TA.

Mobility Allowance

Mobility Allowance is a benefit for disabled people who are unable, or virtually unable, to walk and who are likely to remain in that condition for at least a year. People can receive the allowance whether or not they are working and whether or not they live at home. It is not means-tested, is tax-free, and no National Insurance contributions are needed.

Mobility Allowance replaces the help previously available under the NHS invalid vehicle scheme. However, people who had an invalid vehicle or other benefit from the old scheme can keep it, if they choose, instead of receiving mobility allowance.

ELIGIBILITY

1. **Age**: disabled people aged 5–66 years may claim the allowance. However, 65-year-olds who claim must have been able to satisfy all the conditions before their 65th birthday. If a claim is successful, benefit may be paid up to the age of 75.

2. **Residence**: disabled people must be resident in Great Britain when their claim is made and must have spent 52 weeks during the previous 18 months in England, Scotland, Wales or Northern Ireland.

3. **Disability**: applicants must be so physically disabled that they are unable to walk, or virtually unable to walk, and are likely to remain so for at least a year. This means their ability to walk outside is so limited that it would make very little practical difference if they could not walk at all. An overall assessment of walking ability is based on the following factors: distance; speed; length of time; manner in which the person can walk without severe discomfort.

The person's condition during most of this period must also be such as permits him 'from time to time to benefit from enhanced facilities for locomotion'. In other words, applicants must be physically able to benefit from going out occasionally.

CLAIMING

The claim form is in the Mobility Allowance leaflet (N1.211), available at social security offices. It should be completed and sent to the Mobility Allowance Unit (DHSS), North Fylde Central Office, Norcross, Blackpool, Lancashire, FY5 3TA.

The parents or guardians of children under 16 years of age should complete the form on their behalf and complete the special section at the end of the form. If an adult cannot complete and sign the form himself, another adult (such as an advocate, friend, carer or nurse) should do it for him and explain why on the form.

ASSOCIATED BENEFITS

Mobility Allowance is used by other schemes as a way of confirming physical disablement. The other benefits that mobility allowance beneficiaries may require are as follows:

1. Exemption from vehicle excise duty.
2. Exemptions from VAT when buying motability cars, or car adaptations and other aids.
3. Rate rebates on garages.
4. Inclusion in the Orange Badge Scheme.
5. Driving licences at the age of 16 years.
6. Free medical examination for exemption from the requirement to wear seat belts.
7. Enhanced home insulation grant.
8. British Rail card for disabled people.
9. Severe Disablement Allowance (if of working age and incapable of work).
10. Higher needs allowance in calculating entitlement to housing benefit.

Applications for exemption from vehicle excise duty should be made to the Department of Transport Local Vehicle Licensing Office. They can be made by someone receiving Mobility Allowance, or by a person appointed by the Secretary of State to act on behalf of a Mobility Allowance beneficiary, or by someone nominated by a Mobility Allowance beneficiary (or nominated by the person acting on the beneficiary's behalf). The vehicle must be used solely by, or solely, for the benefit of the Mobility Allowance beneficiary. Beneficiaries can only get exemption for one car. The Mobility Allowance Unit gives details of the application procedure to each person awarded the allowance. Mobility Allowance beneficiaries who do not have exemption should write to the Mobility Allowance Unit. Queries relating to the granting of exemption should be made to the Department of Transport.

Severe Disablement Allowance (SDA)

SDA is given to people who have not been able to work for at least 28 weeks because of physical or mental illness or disability, and who are not entitled to Sickness or Invalidity benefit because they have not paid enough National Insurance contributions. People receiving SDA can be credited with National Insurance contributions. SDA is tax-free, and is not means-tested.

ELIGIBILITY

People who have been incapable of work for at least 196 continuous days (28 weeks) should apply if they meet the following criteria:

1. **Age**: the applicant must be over 16 years of age and under pension age (60 years for women, 65 years for men), but people receiving SDA on the day before they reach pension age can continue receiving it thereafter unless it is replaced by another benefit, such as retirement pension. If the value of this

other benefit is less than the SDA rate, payments of SDA can be made to bring the total amount up to the level of SDA.

People over pension age cannot receive SDA unless they were receiving NCIP, HNCIP or SDA on the day before they reached pension age (or were entitled to it but were receiving an overlapping benefit instead).

Likewise, people over retirement age (65 years for women, 70 years for men) cannot receive SDA unless they were receiving NCIP, HNCIP or SDA on the day before they reached retirement age.

2. **Disability**: incapacity for work is the main qualifying condition for SDA. Applicants must be incapable of work, and they must have been incapable of work for at least 196 continuous days (28 weeks) immediately before the date from which they are claiming benefit. A day when the claimant is in prison or legal custody does not count as a day of incapacity for work.

   Two categories of people can obtain SDA as soon as they become incapable of work, without having to wait 196 days:
   (a) People who have received SDA during the past eight weeks.
   (b) People who used to get SDA (or NCIP or HNCIP) if, during the time since they last had SDA (or NCIP or HNCIP), there have not been any periods of more than eight weeks when they were not signing on as unemployed or receiving a training allowance from an approved training scheme, or getting sickness benefit because of an accident at work. There can be any number of these short gaps between the periods when a claimant is receiving SDA.

The following rules for SDA are extremely complicated and help or advice should be sought from the DHSS office, the local Citizens' Advice Bureau or the local welfare rights organisation in all areas of difficulty. Claims which are based on these rules are referred to as linking claims because they are said to link with an earlier period of entitlement to SDA, NCIP or HNCIP.

80% DISABLEMENT

If a person claiming SDA has been continuously incapable of work for at least 196 days (28 weeks) starting *on or before* his twentieth birthday, he can qualify for SDA on the basis of that incapacity alone. People whose 28-week qualifying period of incapacity for work starts *after* their twentieth birthday must also have been at least 80% disabled throughout the whole of their 28-week qualifying period. There are two exceptions to this rule:

1. Applicants do not have to be 80% disabled if they have

received NCIP, HNCIP or SDA before, or the basis of incapacity for work started on or before their twentieth birthday, and they are making a claim for SDA which links with that earlier period of entitlement.

2.   There is a special rule designed to help people who have only had short breaks in their incapacity for work, but who are not helped by the rules about linking claims. This special rule applies both to people who first claim SDA after the age of 20 but who first became incapable of work before their twentieth birthday, and to people who have already had SDA on the basis of incapacity for work starting on or before the age of 20, but who then have some breaks when they are capable of work. The rule provides that once someone has been continuously incapable of work for 196 days starting on or before his twentieth birthday, he will continue to be treated as having been continuously incapable of work since then provided there are no periods when he is capable of working for more than 182 days (26 weeks). If someone has two or more qualifying periods of incapacity for work starting on or before his twentieth birthday, he does not have to start counting the 182 days (26 weeks) until the end of the latest period. People claiming under this rule do not have to be 80% disabled to qualify for SDA. But unlike people making a linking claim, they have to be continuously incapable of work for at least 28 weeks before they can receive benefit.

CLAIMING

There is an application form in the SDA leaflet (N1.252) available from social security offices. The completed form should be returned to the local social security office (a post-free addressed envelope can be obtained from the post office). If the applicant cannot fill in the form another adult should do it for him and explain this on the form.

Other sources of financial help

Income support

Income Support is a social security benefit to help people who do not have sufficient funds on which to live. It is intended to meet regular weekly needs. People may be able to receive help with exceptional expenses which are difficult for them to pay from their regular income from the Social Fund (see below).

People can obtain help from the Income Support even if they have savings of up to £6,000. If someone has a partner who they are married to, or who they live with as if they were married to them, their partner's savings are counted as well. If savings are worth up to £3,000 it will not influence the Income Support they can receive.

However, savings between £3,000 and £6,000 will make a difference. Each £250, or part of £250, will be treated as if it was bringing in £1.00 a week. If a child has more than £3,000 savings, no allowance will be added on to Income Support for that child. Otherwise a child's savings will not be counted.

The amount of Income Support a person can receive depends mainly on how much the law says they need to live on, and how much money they already have coming in from other sources such as social security benefits and part-time work. Savings worth more than £3,000 will also make a difference.

There are different systems for working out how much Income Support people can receive while living in board and lodging, hostels, residential care or nursing homes. Local social security offices will be able to provide more information about this.

HELP WITH THE COST OF HOUSING

If someone receives Income Support, they will qualify for Housing Benefit from their local council, to help them pay their rent and rates. But they will have to pay part of their rates and water charges themselves. Extra money for any ground rent that has to be paid can also be added to Income Support. Income Support can also help pay the interest on mortgages or home loans. The amount will depend on the person's age.

PEOPLE UNDER 60

If both the person receiving Income Support and their partner are under 60, an amount will be added to cover half the interest that they have to pay for the first 16 weeks after they start receiving Supplementary Benefit or Income Support. After this 16 weeks, an amount to cover all the interest will normally be added on.

PEOPLE AGED 60 OR OVER

If either the person receiving Income Support or their partner is 60 or over, an amount to cover all the interest will normally be added on.

Other benefits

People receiving Income Support do not have to pay for any of the following for themselves, for their partners or for their children:
(a) NHS prescriptions;
(b) NHS dental treatment; and
(c) travel to hospital for NHS treatment.
They will also get help with the cost of glasses and possibly further assistance from the Social Fund if they have a new baby, need to cover funeral expenses or have other exceptional expenses.

For further information about Income Support, leaflet SB20 – A

Guide to Income Support is available from local social security offices.

For advice or help with social security, use Freeline Social Security 0800–666 555 (free telephone enquiry service).

The Social Fund

The Social Fund is a scheme to help people with exceptional expenses which are difficult for them to pay from their regular income. It consists of the following sources of benefit:

(a) Budgeting Loans;
(b) Crisis Loans; and
(c) Community Care Grants.

There is a limited amount of money available for these payments and so when they look at an application, Social Fund officers have to look at the needs of all the applicants and decide which needs can be met from the money available.

BUDGETING LOANS

These are for people receiving Income Support. They are to help them pay for something that they need but which they cannot afford at the time they need it. Savings worth over £500 will influence the right to receive Budgeting Loans.

The loan is usually paid back by taking money from the recipient's social security benefit each week and if they stop receiving benefit, perhaps because they start work, they will still have to pay back the money.

The applicant for the Budgeting Loan, or their partner, must have been getting Income Support for each of the last 26 weeks without a break. One break of 14 days or less does not matter. Their partner is the person who they are married to or the person they live with as if married to them.

People cannot receive a Budgeting Loan if they or their partner are involved in a trade dispute, and the Social Fund officer must be sure that the person can afford to pay the money back.

Application should be made on form SF300: 'Grants and Loans from the Social Fund', available from local social security offices.

CRISIS LOANS

These are to help people pay for things they need urgently because of emergency or disaster. Anyone may be able to get a Crisis Loan. They are not just for people who are getting Income Support or some other social security benefit. But people can only get a Crisis Loan if there is no other way of preventing a serious risk to the health or safety of them or their family. For example, someone might get a Crisis Loan to pay for their immediate needs, if they are burgled and they have no money or savings.

If the recipient is receiving social security benefits, the loan may be paid back by taking money from the benefit each week. If the person isn't receiving social security benefits, the loan will still have to be paid back.

COMMUNITY CARE GRANTS

These are for people receiving Income Support, or who expect to receive Income Support when they move into the community. These grants are to help them:
(a) return to the community rather than be in care ('care' meaning places like hospitals, nursing homes, old people's homes and residential care homes);
(b) return to the community from places like hostels for the homeless, detention centres or local authority care for young people;
(c) stay in the community rather than be in care;
(d) cope with very difficult problems in their family such as disability, long-term illness or family breakdown; and
(e) pay for fares to visit someone who is ill or for another urgent reason.
Savings worth over £500 will influence the right to receive Community Care Grants.

If someone already receives Income Support they will not have to pay back the Community Care Grant. If someone does not receive Income Support when they move into the community they will have to pay the grant back. Applications should be made on Form SF300: 'Grants and Loans from the Social Fund'. This is available from local social security offices.

The following leaflets give information about the Social Fund and other benefits:
FB8: Babies & benefits
FB27: Bringing up children?
FB28: Sick or disabled?
FB29: Help when someone dies.

A detailed explanation of the Social Fund is to be found in leaflet SB16: 'A Guide to the Social Fund'.

All these leaflets are available from local social security offices. The 'phone number and address are in your local 'phone book under 'Social Security' or 'Health & Social Security'. Some of these leaflets will also be available in post offices.

For advice or help with social security use Freeline Social Security 0800-666 555 (free telephone enquiry service).

Vaccine damage payments

There is a scheme which provides a lump sum payment of £20,000 for a person who has suffered permanent and very severe damage as a result of vaccination under a routine public-policy vaccination programme. Further information is available in the DHSS leaflet HB3: 'Payment for Severe Vaccine Damage'.

The Family Fund

The Family Fund is run by the Joseph Rowntree Memorial Trust and is financed by the Government. Its job is to help families caring for a 'severely' handicapped child under the age of 16, by giving a lump sum grant for specific items which arise from the care of the child. Many thousands of families have been helped by the fund. Grants are given by the fund to relieve stress arising from the everyday care of a severely handicapped child. The grants are given for a wide range of needs such as help to purchase a washing machine, clothes, dryers, bedding, a holiday for the family, recreation equipment and help with transport. There is no set list. You should ask for whatever you most need by writing to: Family Fund, PO Box 50, York, YO1 1UY.

Useful addresses for further advice and information

1. Royal Society for Mentally Handicapped Children and Adults (MENCAP), 123 Golden Lane, London EC1Y ORT. Tel: 01-235 9433.
2. Spastics Society, 12 Park Crescent, London W1N 4EQ. Tel: 01-636 5020.
3. Royal Association for Disability and Rehabilitation (RADAR), 25 Mortimer Street, London W1N 8AB. Tel: 01-637 5400.
4. DIAL UK, Dial House, 117 High Street, Clay Cross, Chesterfield, Derbyshire S45 9DZ. Tel: (0246) 864498.
5. Attendance Allowance and Mobility Allowance Unit, DHSS, North Fylde Central Office, Norcross, Blackpool FY5 3TA. Tel: (0253) 856 123.
6. Local DHSS Office. Check telephone directory under: 'Health and Social Security, Department of' for the address and telephone number.
7. National Association of Citizens' Advice Bureaux, 115–123 Pentonville Road, London N1 9LZ. Tel: 01-833 2181 for address of local CAB.
8. DHSS Freephone. Dial 100 and ask for DHSS Freephone for advice on social security benefits.
9. Other advice organisations. There are many organisations which can offer advice, help and information. Check at the local Citizens' Advice Bureau to find out what is available in your area.

CHAPTER 17

Sources of help and advice

James Ross
Formerly Director, Welfare and Counselling Services, MENCAP

In Great Britain we have a massive welfare state system designed to provide support and services, benefits and care for people in need. The real problem for most people is understanding how it works and where to find the help they need. The combined statutory and voluntary agencies which together provide the welfare state services are a tangle of confusing and complicated systems. Most people are confused about who is responsible for various services. Is it a government service? Local authority, voluntary or central Government? Is it social security or social services or the health authority? Where do you go for what? Who is responsible? What am I entitled to? Is it free?

Distinguishing the responsibilities and contributions of the 'professionals' who may be involved in helping people who are mentally handicapped is important because some have access to resources which are independent of the others. The family doctor, for example, has a key role in many of the applications for benefits such as Attendance Allowance and Mobility Allowance, as well as many of the support services necessary for people with a mental handicap.

In this chapter the main sources of help and advice are explained, where to find them and who is responsible for the provision of services or benefits. First it is important to understand the wide range of services provided by central Government, local government (statutory services) and a very large number of voluntary agencies (voluntary services). Some of the main agencies, both statutory and voluntary, are listed at the end of the chapter for easy reference. Details of financial help and social security payments such as Income Support are given in the next chapter.

Health services

The family doctor

For new parents of a handicapped child, the family doctor and the health visitor are the 'key' professionals who can provide, or arrange, the support and help needed. The doctor is the key person who can ensure that you get, or are referred to, the services you need. The existing structure of the health and welfare provision in this country virtually appoints the family doctor as the 'master key' to most of the services, support systems and benefits that people with a mental handicap will require throughout their lives. It is essential to have a family doctor who understands that you may have special needs and who is prepared to provide the care and consideration which may be necessary. (Remember, you can change your doctor at any time.)

In addition to meeting the usual health-care needs for which people visit their family doctor, a GP can recommend a range of other professional support according to the needs of the individual. It is the doctor who 'authorises' appointments for specialist advice or treatment at the hospital, clinic, assessment centre etc. It is the doctor who provides the letter to see a 'specialist' – the consultant who specialises in particular areas of medicine and treatment (paediatrician, psychiatrist, neurologist or psychologist, for example). Families of a mentally handicapped child often need their doctor's recommendation to apply for social services, social security benefits, re-housing and many other services.

The health visitor

Most families will find the health visitor the best source of help and advice, especially in the early days and months of the child's development. She can provide a wealth of information and advice about the local services and also act as the co-ordinator between the various agencies such as social services departments and health authorities. The health visitor, or one of her colleagues called the community nurse, is normally a member of the Community Mental Handicap Team (CMHT) or the District Handicap Team (DHT) which opens up the possibilities for a wide range of supporting services. That is why the health visitor should be looked upon as one of the key workers for help and advice. Of course, as a trained nurse who has undertaken additional specialist training, she is qualified to advise on the care of handicapped babies and young children as well as giving general support to the family. The health visitor can also arrange for special aids, adaptations and other practical support from other departments and voluntary organisations.

Assessment and therapy services

The best source of help in the first place, in getting the advice and treatment you need, is your family doctor, health visitor, school doctor or your local health centre. Parents who suspect that something is not quite right, or are worried about their child's progress, should request a full developmental assessment. This may be carried out by the family doctor or a referral made to a consultant paediatrician or other specialist. If it is found that the child needs special help there is a full range of medical services available. This might include physiotherapy, speech and occupational therapy and/or referral to other specialist consultants.

Primary health care team

Your family doctor, the health visitor and the other community nurses such as the district nurse are part of what is called the Primary Health Care Team. They work closely together and either are based at the health centre or local clinic or are attached to the GP's surgery.

Counselling services

If you need the help of a trained counsellor or help with a particular problem, ask your family doctor for advice. For example, you may want to know about the risk of having another handicapped child. The family doctor will refer you to the Genetic Counselling Clinic which is normally based at one of the local hospitals.

Special aids and equipment

Many items of equipment to help in the care of a disabled person are available through the health services. These include baby buggies (for children over two years), wheelchairs, various items of remedial equipment used in physiotherapy, and aids to feeding and toiletting. If your child is slow to become toilet trained and continues to need nappies by day or night well beyond the usual age, you should ask your health visitor to arrange for a regular supply to be made available.

Health services checklists

The checklists below indicate the services provided by the National Health Service in most districts.

For advice about local health services ask your family doctor or health visitor. Alternatively, information is available at the Citizens' Advice Bureau or the Community Health Council. See the list at the end of the chapter for other suggestions and where to look for advice and information.

PROFESSIONALS

1. Family doctors (GP). ★
2. Health visitors. ★
3. District nurses. ★
4. Community nurses. ★

5. Paediatricians.
6. Psychiatrists.
7. Neurologists.
8. Psychologists.
9. Speech therapists.
10. Physiotherapists.
11. Occupational therapists.
12. Counsellors and specialist advisors.

*Key workers: usually responsible for advising about all the other services and referring to those required.

ESTABLISHMENTS AND SERVICES

1. Hospitals.
2. Welfare centres.
3. Assessment centres.
4. Diagnostic units.
5. Day nurseries.
6. Special residential units.
7. Respite care units.
8. Out-patient clinics.
9. Special care services.

Social services

The social services departments provide a wide range of services for families with a handicapped child. Social workers can offer advice on the many emotional and practical needs of the individual and the family. They may also be able to provide support and counselling during periods of stress. In most social services departments there are social workers who specialise in working with children or adults who are mentally handicapped. They often work closely with the health visitor, community nurse and family doctor to ensure the best possible care and support is given.

Residential care

Local authorities have a statutory duty to provide residential care for both children and adults. Most provide small homes and hostels themselves but an increasing number sponsor places in voluntary and private homes or organise substitute family-type care through fostering or special lodgings schemes.

Respite care is often available for short periods, particularly in cases of emergency (for example, if a mother of a handicapped child has to go into hospital).

Day centres

Day centres are provided by social services departments for people with a mental handicap. They normally go to a day centre at the age of 18 or 19 when they leave school but most local authorities have a special programme to phase-in the change of environment by arranging regular short visits or attendance for one or two days over the first term. Day centres are generally called Adult Training Centres or Social Education Centres but somehow adopt different titles because there is a considerable amount of re-thinking and development of their role.

Parents should ensure that they commence discussion both with the head teacher and the social worker at least a year before their son or daughter leaves school to find out what other opportunities are available in the area. It is a good idea to involve the Education Welfare Officer, the Specialist Careers Advisor and any other professional who has been involved in the past few years.

The main purpose of the day centre is to build on the work that has been achieved at school and to improve the young adult's general and social education and to develop work skills. The manager or the deputy manager will be pleased to explain the centre's programme or discuss any problems. This is best done before the young person leaves school. Parents should remember to ask about further opportunities: what is available following a period of training at the centre? In some areas there are sheltered workshops where the workers are registered disabled and earn proper wages. There are also other work opportunities and schemes being developed which need to be explored. In addition to the day centre manager and staff, the Disablement Resettlement Officer (DRO), who is employed by the Department of Employment, may be able to give further advice and help. Ask at the nearest Job Centre for the name and address of the DRO.

Social services checklist

Table 17.1 provides a checklist of the services provided by local authority social services departments for people with a mental handicap.

Table 17.1 Social services checklist.

Social work support	Social worker★ Specialist social worker
Day services (ATC etc.) – special care	Manager Instructors
Residential services including respite care	Residential social worker
Equipment, adaptations etc.	Occupational therapist

★The social worker is the key worker responsible for advising about, referring to and co-ordinating the other services.

Community Mental Handicap Team

In most areas the District Health Authority and the local authority social services department have established what is called the Community Mental Handicap Team (CMHT). It usually includes a specialist social worker and community nurse and other professionals. The role of the CMHT is to provide specialist help and advice as well as co-ordinating the area's services for people with a mental handicap. The CMHT is a good point of contact for parents and can check whether all the necessary services are being provided.

To find out if there is a local CMHT contact the social services department, your local health authority, or ask your family doctor or health visitor.

Voluntary services

We are fortunate to have a large number of voluntary organisations which provide excellent services and advice. Most of them specialise in particular areas of need and a list of the main ones is given at the end of this chapter.

The Royal Society for Mentally Handicapped Children and Adults (MENCAP) is the national organisation founded by, and for, parents. There are over 500 local MENCAP societies in England, Wales and Northern Ireland, providing a source of advice, help and support for parents. They often act as an umbrella organisation and are able to tell you about all the other services available in the neighbourhood. The Royal Society provides professional support for local MENCAP societies and for individual parents through a network of District Offices, Divisional Offices, and the National Centre in London. MENCAP District Officers are always prepared to help and advise parents. Their telephone numbers can be found in the local directory under 'MENCAP'. They will also give information about the local MENCAP society and advise on who to contact in your area.

Mobility and transport services

These are provided by various organisations and the help available ranges from cash benefits to concessionary fares and ambulance services.

Mobility Allowance

The Mobility Allowance is a non-means tested benefit and is tax-free. It is only given to people between the ages of five and 65 at the time of claiming, who are unable or virtually unable to walk or who would endanger their lives because of the exertion needed to walk. Full details are given in the preceding chapter which covers finance and benefits.

Health and local authority transport

Most local authorities provide door-to-door transport for people who are mentally handicapped attending facilities such as schools and day centres. Some authorities also provide transport for club activities, sports, outings and group holidays. Health authorities provide ambulance services for emergencies, and for out-patient treatment on a doctor's recommendation.

Bus passes

Most local authorities operate a concessionary fares scheme, either free or at a reduced rate, usually by means of a bus pass. Further information will be available at your local council offices.

Rail travel

Services and information about concessionary fares under the Disabled Persons Railcard Discount Travel are available from most British Rail Stations. Ask for the booklet 'British Rail and Disabled Travellers'.

People requiring assistance to make a train journey should telephone to let BR staff know beforehand, i.e., at the station where the journey is to commence. They are usually most helpful.

Local mobility schemes

There are a wide variety of community transport schemes organised by statutory and voluntary organisations e.g. Dial-A-Ride. Details should be available from the local social services department or the local MENCAP society.

Orange badge parking scheme

The 'orange badge parking scheme' is for disabled people who have considerable difficulty in walking or who are blind. You may need a certificate from your doctor unless you are in one of certain categories. If you display the badge in a car you drive, or in one driven for you, you can do the following:

1. Park free, and without limit, at parking meters.
2. Park without time limits in limited-waiting areas.
3. Park for up to two hours on yellow lines, using a special parking disc to show the time the car was parked.

The badges can be used throughout Great Britain, but not in some areas in central London. If you want to know more get the leaflet 'Parking Concessions for Disabled and Blind People' from the traffic department or social services department of your local council.

Local information

In most areas there are voluntary and statutory organisations which provide advice and information. To find out more about them ask at the local library, the local post office or the Citizens' Advice Bureau.

National addresses and telephone numbers

1. DIAL UK
    DIAL House
    117 High Street
    Clay Cross
    Chesterfield
    Derbyshire S45 9DZ
    Tel: (0246) 864498

2. Royal Association for Disability
    and Rehabilitation (RADAR)
    25 Mortimer Street
    London W1N 8AB
    Tel: 01-637 5400

3. Disabled Living Foundation (DLF)
    380/384 Harrow Road
    London W9 2HU
    Tel: 01-289 6111

4. Royal Society for Mentally Handicapped
    Children and Adults (MENCAP)
    123 Golden Lane
    London EC1Y ORT
    Tel: 01-253 9433

5. National Association for Mental Health
    (MIND)
    22 Harley Street
    London W1N 2ED
    Tel: 01-637 0741

6. Spastics Society
    12 Park Crescent
    London W1N 4EQ
    Tel: 01-636 5020

7. Age Concern England
    Bernard Sunley House
    60 Pitcairn Road
    Mitcham
    Surrey CR4 3LL
    Tel: 01-640 5431

8. Association for Spina Bifida and Hydrocephalus
    (ASBAH)
    22 Upper Woburn Place
    London WC1H OEP
    Tel: 01-388 1382

9. British Diabetic Association
    10 Queen Anne Street
    London W1M OBD
    Tel: 01-323 1531

10. British Epilepsy Association
    Crowthorne House
    New Wokingham Road
    Wokingham
    Berkshire RG11 3AY
    Tel: (0344) 773122

11. Association of Crossroads
    Care Attendant Schemes
    94 Coton Road
    Rugby
    Warwickshire CV21 4LN
    Tel: (0788) 73653

12. General Medical Council
    44 Hallam Street
    London W1
    Tel: 01-580 7642

13. Attendance Allowance Unit
    DHSS
    North Fylde Central Office
    Norcross
    Blackpool FY5 3TA
    Tel: (0253) 856 123

14. Mobility Allowance Unit
    DHSS
    North Fylde Central Office
    Norcross
    Blackpool FY5 3TA
    (Letters to Norcross,
    telephone enquiries to
    Warbeck Hill
    Tel: (0253) 52311)

15. Association of Carers
    21–23 New Road
    Chatham
    Kent ME4 4QJ
    Tel: (0634) 813981

16. Wales Council for the Disabled
    Caerbragdy Industrial Estate
    Bedwas Road
    Caerphilly
    Mid Glamorgan CF8 3SL
    Tel: (0222) 887325

17. Scottish Council on Disability
    Princes House
    5 Shandwick Place
    Edinburgh EH2 4RG
    Tel: 031-229 8632

18. The Mobility Information Service
    Copthorne Community Hall
    Shelton Road
    Copthorne
    Shrewsbury
    Tel: (0743) 68383

19. Voluntary Council for Handicapped Children
    (VCHC)
    8 Wakley Street
    London EC1V 7QE
    Tel: 01-278 9441

20. Association of Parents of Vaccine Damaged Children
    2 Church Street
    Shipton-on-the-Stour
    Warwickshire CV36 4AP
    Tel: (0608) 61595

21. Catholic Handicapped Children's Fellowship
    2 The Villas
    Hare Law
    Stanley
    Co Durham DM9 8DQ
    Tel: (027) 34379

22. Children's Legal Centre
    20 Compton Terrace
    London N1 2UN
    Tel: 01-359 6251/2

23. Children's Society, Church of England
    Edward Rudolf House,
    Margery Street,
    London WC1X 0SL
    Tel: 01-837 4299

24. Compassionate Friends
    5 Lower Clifton Hill
    Bristol 8
    Tel: (0272) 292778
    Bereaved parents organization offering mutual friendship
    and understanding.

25. Contact-a-Family
    16 Strutton Ground
    London SW1
    Tel: 01-222 2695

26. Cruse, The National Organisation for the
    Widowed and their Children
    Cruse House
    126 Sheen Road
    Richmond
    Surrey TW9 1UR
    Tel: 01-940 4818

27. Disability Alliance
    25 Denmark Street
    London WC2H 8NJ
    Tel: 01-240 0806

28. Down's Children's Association
    4 Oxford Street
    London W1
    Tel: 01-580 0511/2
    Counselling, early training and education advice for
    families with a Down's syndrome child.

29. Equipment for the Disabled
    Mary Marlborough Lodge
    Nuffield Orthopaedic Centre
    Headington
    Oxford OX3 7LD
    Tel: (0865) 750103

30. Family Fund
    PO Box 50
    York YO1 1UY
    Tel: (0904) 21115

Provides financial help to families caring for a very
severely handicapped child.

31. Family Planning and Information Service
    27–35 Mortimer Street
    London W1N 7RJ
    Tel: 01-636 7866

32. Family Welfare Association
    501–505 Kingsland Road
    Dalston
    London E8 4AU
    Tel: 01-254 6251

33. Home Farm Trust Homes for the Mentally Handicapped
    43/45 Queens Road
    Clifton
    Bristol BS8 1QQ
    Tel: (0272) 23746

34. In Touch Trust
    10 Norman Road
    Sale
    Cheshire M33 3DF
    Tel: 061-962 4441
    Mental Handicap contacts and information service.

35. Jewish Society for the Mentally Handicapped
    Stanmore Cottage
    Old Church Lane
    Stanmore
    Middlesex
    Tel: 01-954 0257/1663

36. Kith and Kids
    27 Old Park Ridings
    Grange Park
    London N21 2EX
    Tel: 01-360 5621
    Self-help group for parents with a handicapped child.

37. Marriage Guidance Council
    Herbert Gray College
    Little Church Street
    Rugby
    Warwickshire CV21 3AP
    Tel: (0788) 73241

38. Motability
    Boundary House
    91–93 Charterhouse Street
    London EC1M 6BT
    Tel: 01-253 1211

39. National Association of Citizens' Advice Bureaux
    110 Drury Lane
    London WC2B
    Tel: 01-836 9231

40. National Association for Deaf, Blind
    and Rubella Handicapped
    311 Grays Inn Road
    London WC1X 8PT
    Tel: 01-278 1000
    Support and advice for families with deaf-blind
    babies, children or young adults.

41. National Autistic Society
    276 Willesden Lane
    London NW2
    Tel: 01-451 3844

42. National Children's Bureau
    8 Wakley Street
    Islington
    London EC1V 7QE
    Tel: 01-278 9441

Further reading

1. *Parents Information Bulletin A–Z* (MENCAP, 1984).
2. *Disability Rights Handbook* (The Disability Alliance, published annually).
3. Bicknell, J., *Right from the Start* (MENCAP, 1981).
4. *Under 5's with Special Needs* (Advisory Centre for Education, 1984).
5. *ACE Special Education Handbook* (Advisory Centre for Education, 1983).
6. *A Summary of the Education Act 1981* (Advisory Centre for Education, 1981).
7. Anderson, D., *Social Work and Mental Handicap* (Macmillan Press Ltd, 1982).
8. Apley, J., *Care of the Handicapped Child* (Heinemann, 1978).
9. Ayer, S., Alaszewski, A., *Community Care and the Mentally Handicapped: Services for Mothers and Their Mentally Handicapped Children* (Croom Helm, 1984).

10. Baldwin, D., *Understanding Your Baby* (NFER, 1983).
11. Bishop, M., Copley, M., Porter, J., *Portage* (NFER, 1986).
12. Brown, R., *Integrated Programmes for Handicapped Adolescents and Adults*, (Croom Helm, 1984).
13. Brown, W., *Practical Guidance for Those Who Work with Autistic Children* (The National Autistic Society).
14. Carr, J., *Helping Your Handicapped Child* (Penguin, 1985, reprint).
15. Cohen, R., Lakhani, B., *National Welfare Benefits Handbook* (Child Poverty Action Group, 1986).
16. Craft, A. & M., *Sex Education and Counselling for Mentally Handicapped People* (Costello, 1983).
17. Craft, M., Bicknell, S., Hollins, S., *Mental Handicap: A Multi-Disciplinary Approach* (Bailliere Tindall, 1985).
18. Craig, M., *Blessings* (Hodder & Stoughton, 1979).
19. Eden, D. J., *Mental Handicap: An Introduction* (Allen & Unwin, 1976).
20. *Guide to the Social Services* (Family Welfare Association, 1986 ed.).
21. Griffiths, M., Russel, P., *Working Together with Handicapped Children* (Souvenir Press, 1985).
22. Hogg, J., Sebba, J., *Profound Retardation and Multiple Handicap* (Vol 1: Development & Learning, Croom Helm, 1986).
23. Hogg, J., Sebba, J., *Profound Retardation and Multiple Handicap* (Vol 2: Development & Learning, Croom Helm, 1986).
24. *Elements of a Comprehensive Local Service for People with Mental Handicap* (Independent Development Council, 1982).
25. *Pursuing Quality* (Independent Development Council, 1986).
26. Inskip, H., *Family Support Services for Physically and Mentally Handicapped People in Their Own Homes* (Leonard Cheshire Foundation, 1981).
27. *An Ordinary Life* (project paper No. 24 'Comprehensive Locally Based Residential Services for Mentally Handicapped People', Kings' Fund Centre, reprinted, 1984).
28. Kirman, B., *Genetic Counselling* (MENCAP, 1981).
29. Ludlow, J. R., *Down's Syndrome: Let's Be Positive* (Down's Children Association, 1980).
30. Lynes, T., *Penguin Guide to Supplementary Benefits* (Penguin 1985, 5th edition).
31. McCormack, A. E., *Sixteen – And Then What?* (Helena Press, 1984).
32. McCormack, A. E., *Coping with Your Handicapped Child* (Chambers, 1985).
33. *MENCAP Holiday Accommodation Guide with 1986 Supplement* (updated annually, MENCAP, 1986).
34. *Report of the ad hoc Leisure Committee to MENCAP* (MENCAP, 1986).

35. *Day Services, Today and Tomorrow* (MENCAP, 1986).
36. *Housing for Mentally Handicapped People* (New Era Housing Association, MENCAP, 1984).
37. Millard, D. M., *Daily Living with a Handicapped Child* (Croom Helm, 1984).
38. McConachie, H., Mittler, P., *Parents, Professionals and Mentally Handicapped People* (Croom Helm, 1983).
39. Pugh, G., De'Ath, E., *The Needs of Parents* (National Children's Bureau, 1984).
40. Robinson, A., *Respite Care Services for Families with a Handicapped Child* (National Children's Bureau, 1984).
41. Sanctuary, G., *After I'm Gone What Will Happen to My Handicapped Child?* (Souvenir Press, 1984, revised 1985).
42. Thompson, L., *Bringing Up a Mentally Handicapped Child* (Thorsons, 1986).
43. Topping, K. J., *Parents as Educators: Training Parents to Teach Their Children* (Croom Helm, 1986).
44. *The Good Toy Guide* (Toy Libraries Association, 1986).
44. Worthington, A., *Glossary of Mental Handicap and Associated Physical Disorders* (In Touch, 1985).
46. Worthington, A., *Useful Addresses for Parents with a Handicapped Child* (In Touch, 1981).
47. Worthington, A., *Coming to Terms with Mental Handicap* (Helena Press, 1982).

All the above books can be obtained from the MENCAP Bookshop, 123 Golden Lane, London EC1Y ORT. Tel: 01-253 9433.

CHAPTER 18

Prospect 2000: or back to the future?

Professor Peter Mittler CBE
Professor of Special Education, University of Manchester

Now that the year 2000 is only 12 years away, what are the prospects for people with a mental handicap? How will the quality of their lives improve in the next 20 years? Are they more likely to attend an ordinary school or college and to learn alongside others who are not disabled? Will they have more opportunities to continue their education and training in integrated settings? Or will there still be 500 special schools and 500 Adult Training Centres?

Will they have more opportunities for choice and decision-making concerning where and how they live and how and with whom they spend their leisure? Will their needs for personal and sexual relationships be better understood and accepted? Are they more likely to have a properly paid job and if not will they be trained for one? Will they live in an ordinary house with whatever support they need? Will they be more accepted by neighbours and by the general public? Will there be fewer objections from the public when they move into a house in the neighbourhood and less name-calling, exploitation and victimisation? Will they have enough money to live on or will they still be as poor as they are today?

Looking back to the landmark of the 1971 White Paper *Better Services for the Mentally Handicapped* (DHSS, 1971), we certainly seem to have come a long way. But we should not allow ourselves to be complacent. Without in any way diminishing what has been achieved, we need to be aware of the dangers ahead; indeed, warning signals are all too apparent in the pages of this book.

How will people with a mental handicap fare in a society that values and rewards wealth creation; a society that seems to be weakening publicly-funded services; a society that is increasingly divided between the rich and the poor, those with jobs and those without, the haves and the have nots?

The priority that mental handicap enjoyed in the 1970s is no longer in evidence; positive official policies can no longer be relied on; other priorities have become more pressing.

Education for children

The year 1971 was also a landmark year because this was when responsibility for the education of children with severe learning difficulties was transferred from health to education authorities, a decision which has without doubt proved an outstanding success. Although improvements have not been seen in all schools, the quality of education in most schools has improved out of all recognition; teachers have developed innovative and successful methods of teaching both individuals and groups; many have worked in partnership with parents and community agencies and four out of every five schools have developed strong working links with neighbouring schools and colleges (Coupe and Porter, 1986; Jowett, Hegarty and Moses, 1988).

The 1980s began with the passing of the 1981 Education Act, hailed as a charter for children and parents. But the 1981 Education Act has not itself greatly increased the quality of education for children with severe learning difficulties and has not led to greatly increased provision for these children in ordinary schools (Mittler and Farrell, 1987). Nor is there much evidence that the Act has fulfilled its promise of being a parents' charter: the House of Commons Select Committee on Special Education, as well as surveys of LEA practice by the University of London Institute of Education (Goacher *et al.*, 1988) and the Centre for Studies in Integrated Education (Rogers, 1986) suggest that information about the Act is not reaching parents, that many are only minimally involved in decision-making and that the wheels of bureaucracy grind exceedingly slowly. Indeed, as Farrell points out in Chapter 4, it is ironic that the law insists that parents must respond to official letters in 15 or 29 days when LEAs can take up to two or even three years to complete a statement and the Department of Education and Science can take months to answer a letter.

But perhaps these are minor problems in comparison with the 1988 Education Reform Act for children with special needs in general and for those with severe learning difficulties in particular. Although some last-minute concessions were made by the Government, and there is still hope that the detailed regulations will preserve the interests of children with special needs, the whole thrust of this Act could bring integration to a halt and reverse such progress as has been made in the past 10 years.

How will children with special needs fare in the national curriculum and in the barrage of tests to assess progress? If they are excluded from some or all of the national curriculum, how does this affect their chances of integration? Will primary and secondary schools welcome children who cannot cope with the curriculum, children who will by definition fail the tests and who are expensive to teach? Will head teachers use their new financial autonomy to admit and support children with special needs when they could be spending their money on priorities more acceptable to the majority of parents? Is it conceivable that grant-maintained schools will welcome children with severe learning difficulties? If they decide to opt out of LEA control, how will they gain access to the LEA's advisory and support services? Even if the DES provides the funds to pay for such services, will the LEA services still be in place and what priority are they likely to give to requests for help from schools which have registered a vote of no confidence in the LEA?

The undermining of the role and influence of LEAs could set back the development of special education by decades, since such improvements as have taken place for children with special needs are due to a large extent to initiatives taken at LEA level. For example, it is LEAs who have developed authority-wide advisory and support services, taken the lead in making assessments and arranging for additional provision.

Community services for adults

The 1970s saw the development of joint care planning teams and the provision of joint funding, as well as many visits by the Development Team whose reports and recommendations were designed to stimulate more effective local services. As a result of these trends, many local and regional plans for the development of locally-based services were drawn up, some even involving collaboration with voluntary organisations such as MENCAP and its local societies. While some plans were implemented, others remained pious hopes and many were forgotten.

At the end of the 1970s, the Jay Committee spelled out the principles on which community services should be built (DHSS, 1979); these were developed in a series of influential 'Ordinary Life' publications from the Kings' Fund and the Campaign for People with Mental Handicap, as well as in the guidelines for service development and evaluation published by the National Development Group and, after its abolition, by the Independent Development Council for People with Mental Handicap.

The beginning of the 1980s was also marked by a new commitment by the Government to make faster progress in bringing long-stay hospital residents from hospitals into community services. The 'Care in the Community' initiative (DHSS, 1981) made it possible to transfer resources from health to local authorities in the form of a 'dowry' to pay for the services needed by each individual. In the North West Regional Health Authority this is currently worth £17,000 a year for every person being resettled within the framework of agreed guidelines (NWRHA, 1982).

Although these Government initiatives have undoubtedly led to an increase in the number of people leaving hospitals, the quality of services provided varies from region to region. In some areas, attempts are being made to draw up individual service plans for each person, based on careful assessment of needs and matched by a commitment on the part of statutory authorities to meet those needs. In other areas, there is very little monitoring of the quality of services or the extent to which individuals' needs are being met. It has not always been possible for local authorities to provide the necessary back-up, with the result that people may be left without social work or home help support or may have nothing to do during the day because of the absence of day service provision (Raynes, Sumpton and Flynn, 1987).

Despite the infusion of NHS funds for the resettlement of long-stay hospital residents, local authorities have not been provided with the resources to provide services for people already in the community. Indeed, the 1980s have seen a substantial reduction in rate support grant and the introduction of rate capping on a large scale. Accordingly, at the beginning of the 1980s, Adult Training Centres and hostels were full, mainly because of lack of throughput and because there was nowhere else for people to go. At the same time, social workers were overwhelmed by the problems of children who were the victims of abuse and by families in distress and difficulty. Once again, people with mental handicap were relegated to a lower priority group.

All this was happening at a time when social workers and social services managers were becoming increasingly aware of how the needs of mentally handicapped people might be met outside institutional and segregated services. In particular, the use of ordinary housing which developed rapidly in the 1980s, depends for its success on the availability of support for residents, particularly from social workers and home helps. While this has been forthcoming in some areas, it has been absent in many others.

In response to a growing concern about the quality of community services, the House of Commons Social Services Committee produced a hard-hitting and clearly written report, highlighting the contrast between the official rhetoric and the day-to-day lives of many people with a mental handicap. In response, the Government appointed Sir Roy Griffiths to conduct a one-man enquiry into community services; his report suggests that social services departments should take the lead in the planning and provision of community services and that they should be funded to do so. Unfortunately, this message is weakened by vague references to the importance of social services departments purchasing 'packages of care' from the private and voluntary sector, without specifying how such provision can be monitored in order to ensure quality of provision which meets individual needs.

Some positive trends

While some of these trends are alarming, more positive developments should also be mentioned in conclusion.

First, we should note the development of self-advocacy and participation, the beginnings of a tendency for people with mental handicap to speak for themselves, to set up societies to provide mutual support and to speak publicly about their situation in an effort to achieve better services and understanding of their needs. More services now have consumer committees; in addition, more community-based groups are being formed (Crawley, 1988).

Although most people with mental handicaps are still congregated together in segregated services and very few have moved from segregated to integrated services, there are more examples of real contacts, e.g. between staff and pupils of special and ordinary schools; between students of Adult Training Centres and further education colleges (e.g. Jowett, Hegarty and Moses, 1988) and between individual people with a mental handicap and ordinary members of the public.

There is evidence of more favourable public attitudes towards disabled people and an expressed willingness to pay more in taxes to meet their needs. Although the public's sympathy is more towards disabled people in general rather than those with a mental handicap, there is nevertheless wide agreement that they should be in the community rather than in residential institutions. The support of the public is clearly the foundation for any improvements in community services. This in turn is reflected in the attitudes and priorities of lay decision-makers such as elected and appointed members of health and local authorities and of Members of Parliament.

Despite the gloomy implications of recent legislation, the Disabled Persons Act (1986) could act as a major catalyst for change. Starting life as a private member's bill by Mr Tom Clarke MP and initially attracting a less than lukewarm response from the Government, a well-organised lobby succeeded in securing government support, resulting in slow but gradual implementation. The Act marks a major advance, since it provides for direct representation by disabled people or their representatives in discussion and decision-making concerning service provision. The Act calls for a more co-ordinated approach to assessment and provision for people leaving special schools and long-stay hospitals and also recognises the rights and needs of carers.

Families have moved much more to the centre of the stage. They have begun to work in closer partnership with professionals but to insist when necessary on their rights to information and participation on a basis of respect and equality (Mittler and McConachie, 1983).

Finally, it is important to stress the positive contribution which can be made by voluntary organisations to the improvement of public attitudes and the development of effective government policy.

MENCAP has greatly increased its influence and its advocacy role; it has sought to influence government and politicians and has itself pioneered some important initiatives, particularly in the field of supported employment. In the last analysis, people with mental handicaps depend on the support of the public and of the politicians whom they elect. Organisations like MENCAP, therefore, spend an increasing amount of energy in public education. It is particularly important that they provide leadership for the general public and in particular for the media in portraying people with a mental handicap in a positive light rather than as pathetic objects of charity.

Like other voluntary organisations all over the world, MENCAP is having to rethink its role and its organisation in preparation for the twenty-first century. It will need to attract younger parents and family members and people with a mental handicap themselves; like other organisations, they will need to strengthen relationships with and between local associations and to develop policies which meet the needs of their members for information and advocacy.

Above all, people with a mental handicap will need continuing vigilance and advocacy if the major advances of the last 20 years are to be preserved and extended in the decades to come.

Further reading

1. Coupe, J., Porter, J., (eds.) *The Education of Children with Severe Learning Difficulties: Bridging the Gap Between Theory and Practice* (London, Croom Helm, 1986).
2. Crawley, B., *The Growing Voice: A Survey of Self Advocacy Groups in Adult Training Centres in Great Britain* (London, Campaign for People with Mental Handicap, 1988).
3. DHSS, *Better Services for the Mentally Handicapped* (London, HMSO, 1971).
4. DHSS, *Report of Committee of Enquiry into Mental Handicap Nursing and Care* (Chair, P. Jay), 2 vols. (London, HMSO, 1979).
5. DHSS, *Care in the Community: Moving Resources for Care in England* (London, HMSO, 1981).
6. Goacher, B., Evans, J., Welton, J., Wedell, K., *Policy and Provision for Special Educational Needs* (London, Cassell, 1988).
7. Jowett, S., Hegarty, S., Moses, D., *Joining Forces: A Study of Links Between Special and Ordinary Schools* (Windsor, NFER/Nelson, 1988).

8. Mittler, P., McConachie, H., (eds.) *Parents, Professionals and Mentally Handicapped People: Approaches to Partnership* (London, Croom Helm, 1983).
9. Mittler, P., Farrell, P., 'Can children with special educational needs be educated in ordinary schools?', *European Journal of Special Needs Education*, vol. 2, (1987), pp.221–236.
10. North West Regional Health Authority, *Services for People Who Are Mentally Handicapped: A Model District Service* (Manchester, NWRHA, 1982).
11. Raynes, N., Sumpton, R., Flynn, M., *Homes for Mentally Handicapped People* (London, Tavistock, 1987).
12. Rogers, C., *Caught in the Act* (London, Centre for Studies in Integrated Education, 1986).

Index